Praise for *Keeping Kids Fit*

"Through the Michael Phelps Foundation, I work to promote healthy, active lives, especially for children. It's very important that children are active, and Len Saunders has spent the last three decades teaching children how to stay active and healthy.

Michael Phelps, 14-time Olympic Gold Medal Champion

"Getting kids active and keeping them healthy is now more challenging than ever. Len Saunders lays out a plan that can assist all parents in their efforts to help their children discover all that sports and exercise have to offer."

Cal Ripken Jr., Baseball Hall of Fame member
and 19-time Major League Baseball All-Star

"Keeping children active motivates them to be healthy in their adult lives. Len Saunders gives a simple blueprint for success that helps kids keep good habits."

Tony Hawk, champion professional skateboarder

"Len Saunders has successfully educated thousands of children and parents on the importance of living a healthy lifestyle. This book is an outstanding reference for parents and educators alike who want to promote better health for our children."

Digger Phelps, Former Head Basketball Coach, Notre Dame
Fighting Irish and ESPN College Basketball Analyst

"I believe an active child will not only be in good health, but will also have high self esteem and confidence. Children are our future, and it is up to us to make sure they are the best they can be. Len Saunders' Project ACES is a major step in this direction."

Vince Carter, Orlando Magic Guard, 8-Time
NBA All-Star, Olympic Gold Medalist

"Making anything fun is the key to success, especially when talking about fitness. That is exactly what Len Saunders has done."

Chris Jakubauskas, Major League
Baseball Pittsburgh Pirates pitcher

"All parents want their children to have long and prosperous lives, and giving children the gift of good health means making wise choices about nutrition, physical activity, sleep and self-esteem. Len Saunders has been a tireless warrior in the fight against childhood obesity and inactivity for decades."

Dr. Felicia D. Stoler, Doctor of Clinical Nutrition,
registered dietician, exercise physiologist and host of
The Learning Channel's "Honey We're Killing the Kids"

"Childhood obesity is a recognized risk factor for the leading causes of illness and death. Given its increasing prevalence, providing parents with strategies to increase physical activity and improve their children's diet is more important than ever. *Keeping Kids Fit* is an invaluable tool to help parents encourage their children to be active and healthy."

Stephanie Navarro Silvera, Ph.D., Assistant Professor,
Health and Nutrition Sciences, Montclair State University

"Parents play a key role in keeping their children healthy and fit. Len Saunders' programs make staying healthy fun and easy."

Bart Oates, three-time National Football League Super Bowl
Champion and four-time Pro Bowl selection

Keeping Kids Fit

A Family Plan for Raising Active, Healthy Children

Len Saunders

LACHANCE PUBLISHING • NEW YORK
www.lachancepublishing.com

Edited by Victor Starsia and Richard Day Gore

Cover design by Stewart A. Williams

Illustrations by Stephan Schmitz

Library of Congress Control Number: 2009939807

Published by LaChance Publishing LLC
120 Bond Street, Brooklyn, NY 11217
www.lachancepublishing.com

This book is available at special discounts for bulk purchases for sales promotions or premiums. Special editions, including personalized covers, excerpts of existing books, and corporate imprints, can be created in large quantities for special needs. For more information, write to LaChance Publishing or email at info@lachancepublishing.com.

Dedicated with love to Julie, Evan and Ryan

Contents

CHAPTER SIX

First Things First: Warm-Ups and Stretching 55

CHAPTER SEVEN

A Week of Family Fitness and Fun .63

CHAPTER EIGHT

Get in the Game: Kids and Sports 87

CHAPTER NINE

The World Is My Workout Buddy:
School and Family Exercise Programs 97

CHAPTER TEN

PART THREE

Your Child's Inner Fitness:

CHAPTER ELEVEN

CHAPTER TWELVE

Foreword

My earliest childhood memories are those of dance classes with my older sister; of wearing that pink leotard and tights and twirling around and around. At age 5, Santa brought my sister and me a trampoline for Christmas that year, and we would bounce for hours on end. It was after we began trying to do flips that my mother decided we needed a little more structure in our lessons. I was soon on to my second sport, gymnastics.

It was only natural for my mother to involve us in physical activities at an early age. She had been raised in a very active household. My grandfather, a Navy veteran, grew up on a working farm where he did a lot of physical labor, as did his parents before him, so he expected his children, my mother included, to be physically fit. Instead of a swing set in their backyard, my mother and her brother had a chin-up bar. They were required to do chin-ups almost every day from the time they were in first grade. In elementary school, my mother would astound her teachers by doing chin-ups on the playground equipment. On weekends, the family would go for drives in the country and Grandpa would stop the car on a country road and have my mom and uncle run a mile or two. These were not jogs but all-out races, with the winner receiving a small prize. My mother's love of physical fitness stayed with her throughout her life. She spent her time swimming, playing tennis, horseback riding and playing softball. In fact, her nickname during her softball years was "The Deer" because even though she was short, she could really speed around the bases!

Growing up in a fitness-minded household instilled in me the idea that I could do or be anything I wanted as long as I worked hard enough. It was through sport and fitness that I found comfort, excitement and success. The first day I walked into a gymnastics gym, there were pits of foam to play in, bars to swing on and a trampoline to jump and flip around on. What more could a child ask for? I didn't see it as exercise or work, for me it was play time!

The years went by and the hours in the gym got longer, but I still enjoyed playing on the equipment. However, I was learning so much more than athletics. I was terribly shy as a child; I never felt like I fit in at school and dreaded being called on in class. In the gym, I felt at home. I was with other girls that enjoyed the same things I did and we all shared the trials and triumphs of competition. I may have been terrified to raise my hand in the classroom, but on the gymnastics floor I became a new person. I was confident in my routines and enjoyed competing and performing in front of an audience. Over the years, that confidence trickled over into all areas of my life. I became more confident in class and had better self esteem. I grew physically stronger over time and, just as important, my psychological and emotional strength grew as well.

Who would have thought that this once shy child, who was intimidated by everything around her, would grow up to compete in front of millions of people, host a television show and enjoy public speaking? Without gymnastics—without the love of physical activity instilled in me at home—none of it would have been possible.

Of course, you don't have to be an Olympic champion or win the Super Bowl to benefit from physical fitness. Physical fitness provides strength, flexibility, stamina, coordination, body awareness and discipline that can last a lifetime. It can help with anxiety and depression, increase self-esteem, improve a child's self-image, and help kids cope with stress. It can even help kids get better grades. What's more, sports and fitness teach tremendous life lessons such as perseverance, goal setting and good sportsmanship.

I share Len Saunders' concerns about childhood obesity and getting kids to be active beginning at an early age. Today, an estimated one third of all children in the United States are overweight. This epidemic has led to a wide incidence of heart disease, asthma, hypertension and type II diabetes. Like Len, through the Shannon Miller Foundation I am dedicated to fighting this terrible problem.

As a new mother, I want more than anything for my son to be healthy and happy. I know that helping him be physically active from an early age will further these goals. This means less television and more outside and interactive play time. It means talking about good nutrition and a well balanced diet. It means taking a stand for the health and well-being of my child.

Keeping Kids Fit is a tremendous guide for all parents who want their children to be fit and healthy. With down-to-earth advice and ideas for creating healthy habits, this book is a must for every parent, grandparent, coach and teacher. With Len's help, we can all help ensure that our kids are healthy and happy throughout their precious lives.

Shannon Miller
7-time Olympic and 9-time
World Champion Medalist

Introduction

Years ago, when I was a relatively new physical education teacher, I met two people who would change my life. The first was a student of mine named Gregory and the second was the famous NFL football coach George Allen, who was then Chairman of the President's Council on Physical Fitness and Sports.

Overweight and suffering from mild cerebral palsy, Gregory had come to me wearing a leg brace and "Coke bottle" eyeglasses. It soon became clear that gym class might as well have been torture, as far as he was concerned. I began working with Gregory one-on-one during my lunch breaks on things that most children take for granted, like walking and climbing the stairs. I also began having monthly conferences with his parents to ensure that Gregory was eating right and exercising at home. At first, his rest breaks far outweighed his periods of activity. But he kept at it.

Over time, Gregory began to lose weight. Walking the stairs became easier for him. Those rest breaks tapered off and eventually ended. Gregory's self-confidence increased, and he actually started to participate in physical education class. The other children saw his new look, felt his new-found confidence and started showing him the respect he deserved. By the time he graduated, Gregory was a lean, fit kid. He walked so well no one would have guessed that he wore a leg brace. Losing weight, eating well and exercising daily had made a huge difference in Gregory's life.

And that's when George Allen entered the picture. He'd been all over the news claiming how the children in the (former) Soviet Union were far more physically fit than the children in the United States. When I looked at Gregory and saw how far he'd come, I couldn't help but take Mr. Allen's statements personally. Gregory was a perfect example of what can be accomplished with the right motivation, dedication and teachers and parents who care. I just *knew* that if he could get fit, other children could, too and no amount of telling them that they were out of shape compared to kids in another country would motivate them to change. In fact, I felt that kind of negativity was doing more harm than good. So one day, after reading another article by Mr. Allen on the state our children's fitness, I'd had enough. I picked up the phone and called him.

The secretary answered and I said, "This is Len Saunders, may I speak to George, please?" She asked if I meant George Allen, and I said, "Yes." Hoping she wouldn't ask if he knew me—because we were complete strangers—I then said, "He'll know what this is in reference to." A minute passed, but it seemed like forever as I waited for his secretary to come back and tell me to get lost. Finally, though, I heard his distinguished voice:

"Hi Len, this is George. How may I help you?"

I told him that my students and I were very upset over his comments about American children being out of shape. I was nervous at first, but soon the words were tumbling out to the NFL legend. I told him about Gregory. I told him that I believed there were positive ways to motivate kids to take control of their fitness and health and that as a physical education teacher I was determined to make it happen. I knew he might cut me off at any moment so I kept riding my high horse until I was practically out of breath. I ended by promising him that my children would prove him wrong. There was a long pause. Then he amazed me by saying, "You know what, Len, I like your nerve. You have some real backbone." We talked for a few moments more, said goodbye, and that was that.

But it wasn't. A few days later, I received a call at my school. It was George Allen, this time calling me! We spoke again about American children and how he'd like them to be more physically fit. He told me about his trip to the Soviet Union, and how impressed he had been with their ability to get their children in great shape. He then told me he thought I would be a perfect candidate to represent the United States in a fitness exchange with the USSR. He wanted a handful of American schools to take the USSR youth fitness test, while a handful of USSR schools would take the U.S. youth fitness test. Of course I was up to the challenge, and so were my kids. Together we did prove Mr. Allen wrong and he was just as happy about it as we were.

Soon, the *New York Times* was at our school and printed an article about it. More media attention followed, and before I knew it, Project ACES and PACES Day (which you'll read about in this book) were internationally recognized. And it all started with one kid, Gregory, who had the gumption—and the right guidance—to make a difference in his own life.

My job has brought me into contact with thousands of wonderful kids like Gregory in whose lives I have been proud to have made a positive impact. My dedication to making a difference has carried me to the White House to meet President George H. W. Bush and the First Lady, Barbara Bush. It's taken me to a fitness summit at the invitation of Arnold Schwarzenegger, who was at that time Chairman of the President's Council on Physical Fitness and Sports. But the work that I began when I got out of school, helped Gregory and made that call to George Allen is far from over. It's clear that there's a looming crisis in our children's health and fitness, one that's much bigger than anything I can handle on my lunch hour, or address on a segment on CNN. Over many successive Septembers, I've watched as incoming classes have arrived at schools—both the one in which I work and others—in which the kids are less are becoming less physically able to jog around the track and who struggle to perform the warm-up drills that are a standard part of my physical education program.

As today's headlines attest, the childhood obesity and fitness problem is not something that only physical education teachers have observed. The statistics on kids' health are downright frightening. A recent study by the American Heart Association[1] found that fully one third of American children and adolescents are overweight or obese. It also found that most overweight children have at least one additional major physiological risk factor for cardiovascular disease, such as high cholesterol, high triglycerides, high insulin or high blood pressure. It's outrageous—in fact, it's a national shame—that our children's life expectancies may turn out to be shorter than our own.

I'm trying to do what I can to fix this problem. Keeping kids physically fit is not complicated. As with anything worth doing, it just takes time, effort and dedication.

As the cultural, economic and technological environments change, so must our approach to maximizing our kids' health and well-being. Twenty or thirty years ago, children walked to school and played outside without parental supervision. These taken-for-granted aspects of a healthier lifestyle are vanishing, if they are not already gone, so we need innovative methods to make certain our kids don't languish on the couch. Teaching kids

---

[1] American Heart Association Childhood Obesity Research Summit, *Circulation*, April, 2009;119:2114–2123.

that "playtime" is something that takes place sitting down while "mealtime" takes place on the run does them a great disservice.

Most kids have an innate love of active play. My thirty years working with children of all levels of fitness and motivation have made me adept at engaging kids of all ability levels, overcoming their resistance to physical activity and making them feel strong, able and healthy. I've created dozens of children's fitness programs that have successfully motivated millions of children to exercise, and I share them here. This book offers what I believe parents need most: a comprehensive yet easy-to-follow, field-tested toolkit to help ensure the health of their children now and for the rest of their lives.

I believe very strongly that in the same way we work hard to make certain our kids are literate, we must work hard on instructing them in the basics of health and wellness and not simply hope that they will pick it up in school.

Keeping Kids Fit will show you how.

In Part One, Getting Kids Active and Healthy...and Keeping Them That Way!, you'll learn how to partner with your children to motivate them to break the bad habits that lead so many into sedentary, unhealthy lifestyles. You'll learn how to instill good, healthy habits in them and to keep the bad ones from taking hold in the first place. These chapters will help you understand your child's unique psychology as it pertains to fitness and sports so you can choose the right activities to keep your child engaged in maintaining his or her own well being.

Part Two, The Action Plan for Keeping Kids Fit, will show you how to put this information into action. You'll learn how to choose the right exercises for your children and how to do them safely. We'll discuss how to keep fitness fun for the whole family, from healthy indoor activities for rainy days to innovative and exciting programs your child can participate in at school. On every page you'll find simple ways to make fitness not only fun for your children, but, just as important, lasting. The programs described in these pages will give your children a foundation for a healthy life well beyond their childhoods.

Part Three, Your Children's Inner Fitness: Nutrition, Hydration and Sleep, makes these vital topics easy to understand and integrate into your children's total health. You'll learn how to overcome the obstacles to your children's good nutrition and come away with an understanding of how healthy foods can be made just as tempting as the sugary junk that surrounds kids every day. You'll also learn how to get your kids off the computer and into bed for an all-important good night's sleep. I give you easy and fun recipes for healthy snacks, as well as healthy meals, that you can make at home and that your kids will love.

I often think of the expression "baby steps," when it comes to our children's health. Parents need to think big, but start small, and move at a pace in tune with their children's fitness and motivation. I've watched as many parents change the world for their children in a positive way by taking my advice on getting and keeping their kids fit.

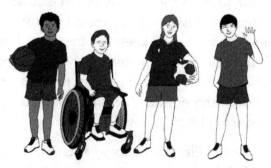

Teach your children lifetime skills which will benefit them now and in the future.

I know firsthand that it's possible to motivate kids to become healthy and fit and for them to grow into healthy, fit adults. I often think back on Gregory, who made such great strides with me all those years ago. George Allen said I had backbone to call him out of the blue, but Gregory was really the one with backbone. He was an inspiration to me as well as to everyone who knew him. It seems to me that all children have a bit of Gregory in them, and I see his spirit reflected in many of the kids with whom I work. With proper guidance, support and good role models, a healthy lifestyle and its benefits are possible for any child, just as they were for Gregory. This book shows you how to get there. Enjoy.

Acknowledgments

I had the distinct pleasure of working with an incredible group of doctors, nutritionists, professors, educators and fitness experts during the writing of this book. They devoted their valuable time to *Keeping Kids Fit*, providing a wealth of information and sharing their wisdom through phone calls, interviews, emails and reviews of the manuscript. I was extremely impressed with their professionalism and their generosity.

Dr. Stephen Rice, who reviewed the chapter on hydration, was very generous with his encyclopedic knowledge of the subject. It means a great deal to me that someone of his stature would take the time to assist in the writing of this book.

The assistance of nutrition experts Linda Mitchell and Susan Patla with the chapter on nutrition was invaluable. "Batting cleanup" for that chapter was Dr. Felicia Stoller, who checked the basics while enhancing the chapter with additional material. Dr. Stoller was also a tremendous help in reviewing the chapter on childhood obesity, her area of expertise for which she is nationally recognized through her television program on The Learning Channel. She is also one of the most inspiring people I have ever met.

The chapter on the benefits of sleep benefitted from the attention of a pair of accomplished professionals: Dr. Vipin Garg, an expert in the field of sleep disorders and sleep medicine, and the well respected pediatrician Dr. Henry Shih.

New information on children and dieting comes in daily, which made the preparation of that chapter a challenge. Luckily, two highly qualified individuals in the field rose to the challenge. Marilou Rochford of Rutgers University and Dr. Stephanie Silvera, both of whom have extensive backgrounds in the area, shared their expertise, and for that I am very grateful.

I was very fortunate to have one of my mentors, Dr. James McCall, review the chapter on sports. Dr. McCall is a highly accomplished expert on physical education and has been very influential in my own life. To include him on this project was a thrill for me. Nicole Astrella, a certified personal trainer with a vast background in children's fitness, did an excellent job reviewing the chapters on exercise, and Dr. Milford Panzer was also of immense help on the topic of exercise.

Rounding out this dream team was Dr. Jamie Leizer, who reviewed the chapters on creating good habits and the psychology of physical activity. A friend for many years, she is well-versed in her field and has extensive experience working with children and sports.

Special thanks as well to everyone else that helped make this book a reality, including Jessica Papin of Dystel and Goderich Literary Management, Cal Ripken Jr., John Maroon, Greg Clifton, Michael Phelps, Tony Hawk, David Ratner, Susan Intile, Digger Phelps, Stephan Schmitz, David Abramson, Chris Jakubauskas, Michael Sciavolino, Dr. Kristen Williams, Sam Elowitch, HJ Saunders, The Youth Fitness Coalition, Inc. and Victor Starsia and Richard Day Gore at LaChance Publishing.

PART ONE

Getting Kids Active and Healthy... and Keeping Them That Way!

CHAPTER ONE

The Childhood Health Crisis

Childhood obesity is on the rise. More and more children are developing what once was known as adult-onset diabetes, a condition—as its name implies—that was once believed to affect only grownups. Physical education and recreation programs are being reduced in your town and across your state. To add insult to all of this injury, we know to our chagrin that our kids already lead fairly sedentary lives; for many parents, the idea of sending them outside to play until dinner is unthinkable, as quaint and outmoded an idea as the one-room schoolhouse. Moreover, we live in the age of technology, where games are virtual, where "playing" may involve nothing more than moving one's fingers and physical exertion is non-existent. This is a deadly trend.

The Surgeon General reports that the prevalence of overweight children has more than doubled in the past 20 years.[1] Heart disease is still the number one killer in the United States and the data shows that most overweight children will grow up to be

---

[1] *The Surgeon General's Call to Action to Prevent and Decrease Overweight and Obesity*, January 11, 2007.

overweight adults, at increased risk not only for heart disease, but also type 2 diabetes, stroke, certain kinds of cancer and osteoarthritis. The declining overall health of our children is a problem that has grown along with their waistlines, and there is no immediate solution in sight.

Unfortunately, there is no one reason for this crisis; it's the sum of many factors. Every year, there seem to be fewer ways for kids to maintain the active lifestyle that was once believed to be a natural part of childhood. When I was a child, I walked home two miles from elementary school every day and then went outside and played until dinnertime. In most neighborhoods, this doesn't happen anymore. Parents are understandably afraid to allow their children outside to play by themselves, and walking to and from school unaccompanied by an adult is often out of the question; in fact, many school districts now prohibit children from walking to school. In many households, both parents are employed and may not have as much time to spend with their children as they would

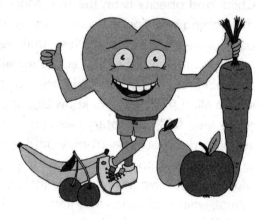

Parents play a key role in keeping their children healthy!

like. Often, children must stay in their homes after school or spend time at a daycare facility. In both cases, most children tend to be sedentary until their parents arrive on the scene. Once they experience sustained forms of inactivity, negative health habits may develop, which bring with them long-term negative health consequences.

fering a greater selection of healthy items while lowering the fat content of some of their meals. This is a step in the right direction, but a child's guardian is still well advised to try to monitor everything a child eats, even foods that are billed as "lite" or "healthy choices."

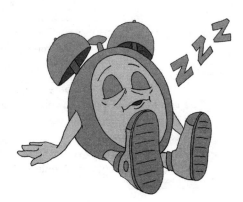

Parents must lead by example. Kids are like mirrors, reflecting back the behaviors they witness daily. Since poor eating habits and sedentary lifestyles are widespread among many adults, children who see this behavior as the norm will most certainly imitate it. For ex-

There's no time like the present to teach children about being healthy. You snooze… they lose!

ample, adults should avoid engaging in non-acceptable behaviors around their children, such as smoking. Smoking cigarettes around children not only makes them believe that it's acceptable behavior, but also exposes them to second-hand smoke which can cause respiratory problems (such as asthma) in children and may impact their cardiovascular disease risk over their lifetimes.

Adults don't have to be perfect, but it's clear that when children see their parents make an effort to eat a healthy, wholesome diet, get enough sleep and exercise daily, they grow up believing it's important and will imitate those behaviors. In cases where a physical disability or illness prevents a parent from leading by example, a parent can still be verbally supportive of their children. Motivate him or her to perform and cheer on any effort your child makes. Positive reinforcement means a lot to a child when performing any task. You can remember your responsibil-

Figure 1.1 *Essential C's in the aCtivity Model of Success!*

A**C**tivity:
Creativity
Commitment
Concern
Communication
Conditioning

As a parent or guardian:
Be **creative** about getting your child involved in **activity**.
Be **committed** to getting your child involved in **activity**.
Be **concerned** about your child's progress in that **activity**.
Be **communicative** to your child about being involved in **activity**.
Be educated about **conditioning** your child through **activity**.

ities for your child's health by using the "aCtivity model" of success (Figure 1.1).

It's interesting to talk in general about the health problems facing our youth. But what everyone really wants to know is, how is my child being affected? Let's find out where your child fits in. Figure 1.2 is a simple quiz to see if your child is leading a healthy lifestyle. It will give you an idea of how your child rates among all kids. Just place a check mark in the appropriate column, and then put the corresponding point total in the far right column. When you've answered all of the questions, tally the points and put your grand total in the bottom right. The highest point total is 55 (If you score 55, you should be writing this book!)

If your score is below 30 points, or even if you have scored within the average, you need to start thinking seriously about making some changes. Think about what you can do to make your child score higher on this test. Will you teach your child to enjoy a new, healthier lifestyle, or will you give in to the unhealthiness of modern society? The answer is easy: do what is

Figure 1.2

Scoring Key

5 points = 5 to 7 days a week   3 points = 3 to 5 days a week   1 point = 2 or fewer days per week

	Daily/ Often 5 Points	On Occasion 3 Points	Rarely or Never 1 Point	Points
How often is your child physically active?				
How often does your child have physical education class?				
Do you involve your child in local recreation activities?				
How often do you walk with your child to school or take family walks?				
How often do you limit your child's television time?				
How often do you limit your child's computer time?				
How often do you limit your child's video game time?				
How often does your child drink 8 oz. of water each day?				
How often do you engage in physical activity with your child?				
How often do you consider yourself a proper role model for your children?				
How often do your children consume servings of fruits and vegetables each day?				
How often does your child get at least 8 to 10 hours of sleep at night?				
Totals				
Grand Total				

50–60 Points—Your child has an excellent healthy lifestyle
40–49 Points—Your child has an above average healthy lifestyle
30–39 Points—Your child has an average healthy lifestyle
Below 30 Points—Your child has a below average healthy lifestyle

best for your child's health. Below I list ten ways you can begin taking steps to lower your child's risk of serious long-term health problems. We'll take a closer look at all of these suggestions throughout this book.

Len's Top Ten Surefire Tips for Keeping Kids Fit

1. **Get Involved.** You must take an active role in your children's fitness. Create time each day for your children to exercise and initiate active play.

2. **Explain the Bank Method.** Do you think your children understand the immediate and long-term benefits of fitness when you tell them to exercise? Most young children are not interested in exercise because they don't comprehend the reasoning behind all the work. Introduce the "bank method" when discussing exercise. Explain that the deposit you make now gives you confidence even when you aren't using it and it will be there in the future when you need it. It's the same with exercise. Each new health deposit will pay dividends in the future.

3. **Educate Your Kids about Getting and Keeping Fit.** Your kids will be more likely to take an interest in their own health if they understand the "what's and why's" of nutrition and fitness and how these principles apply to them now and in their future. This vital information is found later on in this book.

4. **Lead by Example.** Simply put, you won't be taken seriously unless you lead by example. You'll have a hard time convincing your child not to smoke if you smoke. The same goes for healthy eating.

5. **Recognize That as a Parent You Must Adapt to the Times.** If your community isn't as safe as the one you grew up in, you must make time to go out and play with your

children or take turns with a neighbor to assure that there is adequate supervision during outdoor play.

6. **Treat Exercise as Daily Nourishment.** Just as eating is part of a child's daily routine, make exercise part of the daily routine. A little exercise is better than none.

7. **Use Less Technology.** One of the major challenges parents face is the widespread use of technology among children. Do what you can to have your children exercise more than just their thumbs for texting and their hands on the game controller.

8. **Support Daily, Quality Physical Education.** With physical education programs being cut in schools, parents must fight to keep their children healthy. Talk to your child's school board and let them know that PE is a vital part of your child's overall education.

9. **Support Your Local Recreation Department.** Municipal recreation programs are also feeling the budget crunch. Show support for your local recreation department. Don't hesitate to contact your local government officials and express your displeasure with the health and PE programs available to your child. Let them know you want more of both. Discuss ways of improving the funding for your local programs. You cannot do it alone, so recruit other neighbors with the same interests to join in the fight.

10. **Watch the Liquid Intake.** It sounds so simple, but it's so important because 1 in 5 calories consumed by children comes from liquids. Reducing the sugary drinks children consume is a great start in fighting childhood obesity or being overweight.

Okay, we've looked at some of the challenges that face us as a society, as families and as individuals on the issue of children's health. We've examined ways you can assess how these issues might be impacting your kids. You've learned some innovative ways to look at exercise and fitness that will make it easier to integrate wellness into your children's agenda.

Remember those 10 tips for keeping kids fit? Let's learn more about how to put them to use. Read on.

CHAPTER TWO

Motivating Kids to Be Active

Showing leadership in getting your kids eating right, exercising regularly and having other good health habits is critically important to keeping your kids fit. But just how do you go about motivating your child to develop and to maintain great fitness habits? To find out, we need to answer two questions. First, what motivates kids to enjoy physical activity? Second, what discourages kids from enjoying physical activity?

In this chapter, we'll get into the minds of children and find the answers. We'll go over suggestions for reducing the anxiety and stress that is sometimes associated with physical activity by children. We'll look at the arguments for and against competition as a motivator, and whether measuring your child's progress against his or her peers is a good recipe for success. I will give you some tips on how to get kids to enjoy sport and exercise that I have found work wonders with just about every kid. Finally, I'll give you proven methods for reducing the general stress and anxiety that might be negatively impacting your childrens' motivation and health. Ready? Let's go!

Is Competition Good for Children?

Competition is usually a contest, where a winner is selected from among two or more opponents. Some children, particularly those who have had success in competitive sports, thrive on competition. For others, competition can sometimes cause hostility, passivity, or extreme sensitivity. Among parents and professionals who deal directly with children's physical fitness, there are generally two competing views on the subject of competition. One view is that competition is healthy, as it prepares children for the "real world" which is filled with winners and losers. When a responsible adult closely monitors competition, it can encourage excellence and build character and self-esteem. Schools should teach students how to handle winning and losing, instead of protecting them from such valuable experiences.

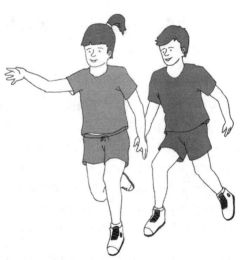

What motivates your children to be active?

On the "anti-competition" side, one most often hears the argument that competition leads to hurt feelings and diminished confidence. It makes children hostile and angry, setting up a situation that could prove to be dangerous to some children. It is a form of bullying, where many children are ostracized for their lack of skills. Schools and clubs should offer only activities in which all students can feel comfortable and important, not threatened.

What is your view? I believe that sport and exercise do prepare children for the real world by teaching habits of physical activity that can last a lifetime. However, *unhealthy* competition, where winning and losing and beating the other competitor take precedence over everything else, has no positive impact on your child's future, and in many cases can be detrimental. Usually, the small number of children who win on a regular basis or have higher athletic skill levels love competition. But the vast majority of kids who lack these skills fear it, with the result that large numbers of kids are turned off to exercise for life. Most of the time, it's because children who consistently lose get bored, embarrassed, and unfavorably compared to children who are more "successful." In fact, some schools have eliminated competition completely from the curriculum and in many other schools there is much less emphasis on competition and much more on teaching lifetime skills, teamwork, safety, and giving one's best effort.

If kids experience failure on a regular basis, they will be turned off to physical activity. In some cases, this encourages kids to gravitate towards sedentary activities, which often leads to a generally unhealthy lifestyle. How do parents motivate kids who have been conditioned to dislike physical activity due to poor instruction, undeveloped skills, and a history of failure? Parents need to turn negative experiences into positive experiences creatively and constructively. For example, if a child strikes out in a baseball game, the focus should not be on making the out, but on the child's effort, or the quality of his form while swinging the bat. Praise will encourage confidence the next time around.

The question of whether competition is good for children is not an easy one. I believe the answer is really both yes and no. Before you say, "huh?" let me explain by quoting the old adage, "different strokes for different folks." In simple terms, different people like different things. Competition can be good for some, but bad for others. It is good if your child succeeds, but bad if your child does not succeed. As parents, we are extremely proud of our children when they are successful at something. We see the positive impact it is making in their lives, but often do not truly realize the negative impact it may be having on another child's life. Is there an alternative, one that could be considered "healthy" competition for most children? There is, and we'll examine *individualized competition* and its positive effect on our children.

Healthy Competition

Over 25 years ago, I had an extraordinary child in class who was confined to a wheelchair but had an almost encyclopedic knowledge of sports. He was mainstreamed into a class of extremely nice, sensitive and compassionate kids who would bend over backwards to help him, which help he never accepted. He was "Mr. Independent."

As the year progressed, I got to know him better and my respect for him grew. He did whatever he was physically capable of doing in every activity. If the class played whiffle ball, he would get up like every other child, swing at a pitch, and wheel his chair to first base. If the other team took it easy on him, he loudly let them know he did not want any special privileges. He was truly remarkable.

One day he confessed to me how upsetting it was for him to compete with the other children. He said, "There is no way I can ever compete with the rest of the class. I'm at such a big disadvantage. I can never measure up to their skills." I was, frankly, stunned by his admission, and there was long, awkward silence, while I tried to find something to say. You see, this child had been my inspiration, and his words struck me as if I had just heard that my favorite superhero was giving up. I could see his eyes were beginning to well up with tears, and my heart broke.

Finally, I looked him squarely in the eyes and said, "Who says you have to compete with them?" There was another silence, and I could see that he was thinking it over. He then replied with one word: "Understood." From that point on, he was still the same motivated child, but it seemed as if the weight of the world had been lifted off his shoulders.

Lesson learned...by me! I learned more about competition among children that day than I had in all my years at college. From that point on, I knew I had to figure out how to get kids to realize that the best competition occurs when they try to achieve their *personal best*. I believe that individualized competition is the answer.

Individualized Competition

With individualized competition, your child competes with only one person: himself! Where regular competition pits one child against another, producing a winner and a loser, individualized competition eliminates the loser.

Think of it this way: your children take many tests in school, whether in math, science, language or physical education. What is the first thing most kids do when they receive their score back from the teacher? Compare notes. But there are always some kids who don't announce their grades. Do you know why? Of course: their grades may be low enough to cause embarrassment and be a hit to their self-esteem.

It's the same with physical activity. Suppose a PE class is asked to take a fitness test that includes completing as many pushups as possible in a given time. Johnny is able to perform 50 pushups in a minute, but Sally, who knows about Johnny's score, manages only 5 pushups in the allotted time. Should she feel good or bad about her performance? In my view, if Sally gave it her best, she should be proud of her accomplishment. In other words, Sally must compete against herself, not Johnny, since the differences in the two children's body composition, skills and innate strength make any comparison between them a false one. Sally needs to look at *her own* performance only, and build on it. So the next time she tries to do as many pushups as she can in one minute, she does not try for 50, but rather for 6 pushups, an admirable increase on her previous score. Once *realistic* goals are set, children will set higher standards for themselves.

The concept is easily applied to organized sports. Suppose Sally and Johnny are both playing in a recreational basketball game. Sally plays an all-around better game, scoring 20 points and 10 rebounds, while Johnny scores no points and no rebounds. It may be that she is just more skilled in basketball, while Johnny has a harder time at it. Again, Johnny knows how successful Sally was in the game, and comparing his own performance to hers may affect his self-esteem, and he may shy away from playing basketball in the future.

But what if Johnny set realistic goals for himself, and didn't compete with Sally's successes? What if Johnny set the following personal goals:

- Try to make a basket.
- Try to get a rebound.
- Get an extra pass.
- Get an extra assist.

As long as Johnny is not trying to equal Sally's output, he is more likely to reach his own goals. *Attainable goals have a much higher frequency of success,* and they give a child something easier to build on thereafter. Reaching one's goals is not easy, however; it takes work, and children need to practice their skills at home with a parent to help attain their goals. There is no magic involved when you try to improve on a past performance; practice does make perfect. Practice also promotes family time, when the parent and child can work together on enhancing skills. Success in most activities often becomes a matter of how much a child wants to achieve it. How different children get there varies, as they each encounter different obstacles, expectations, and guidance. Remember, children may not always steadily improve on their own personal best, but trying for improvement through honest effort is a victory in itself.

It's up to you to decide how you feel about competitive versus non-competitive activities. However, regardless of what you decide, in my experience the factors that motivate kids to stay with fitness are the same. Here are the top 10 ways that I have found work best in motivating kids to enjoy physical activity.

Len's Top Ten Tips to Motivate Kids to Be Active

1. **Give Kids the Opportunity to be Active.** Take the time to play with your children. Five minutes here, 10 minutes there makes all the difference. Try to plan family walks when you can, and even though it may be sedentary, watch ballgames on television with your children, as it builds interest in a physical activity. During the game, every time a commercial comes on, exercise with your children (more on this later). Be a physical activity leader, not a physical in-activity leader.

2. **Get Friends Involved.** Try to sign up your child for activities with his or her friends. Make a few phone calls to the parents of your child's friends to see if there is interest. Once you have them playing together, try to carpool with the other kids, and perhaps take it a step further, by taking the kids out for a healthy snack when the activity is over. Strong bonds of friendship mean the world to children, and this little extra effort will be an enormous help in motivating your child to stay with an activity.

3. **Choose the Right Activities.** Sometimes, children are placed in the wrong activity. If your child is shy or timid, aggressive sports like football may not be right for her, or if your child is not particularly fast, track may not be the best activity. Place your child in an activity you know she will be comfortable with, and take into account her personality, skills, size and desires. Select an activity in which she may experience some success. Talk to your child to find out what activity excites her, and try to build on that excite-

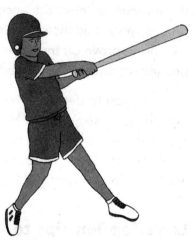

Choose activities that are right for your children.

ment. As an added benefit, you may find out something new that you never would have known about your child.

4. **Make Fun the Focus.** For many kids, as soon as the focus of an activity becomes "being the best" or winning all the time, much of the fun, and a good deal of interest, are lost. Find an activity that is enjoyable to your child, one with the right type of leadership from a coach, teacher, or mentor. Teach your child to always give his best effort, and to be proud of his accomplishments. Teach him to strive to be the best he can be, and always compliment his efforts.

5. **Rebalance the Competition-to-Fun Ratio.** Competition versus fun: guess which should weigh more on the scale? Winning is fine, but is should never outweigh the joy of simply participating in a physical activity.

6. **Teach Kids the Health Benefits of Physical Exercise.** Whether they are playing sports or just doing calisthenics, children should understand that the activity is helping them

to stay healthy. Talk to your children about the health benefits of their activities For example, if your child is on the track team and participates in the mile run, compliment his performance in the race, and mention that running improves his cardiovascular and muscular endurance. Explain how he is making his heart stronger and improving his ability to run further and faster.

7. **Teach Kids that Physical Activity Improves Cognitive Skills.** It is now well-established that exercise and physical activity lead to improved brain function. Exercise can, in fact, create a stronger, faster brain. Tell your kids that every form of exercise they do causes more blood to travel to the brain which in turn helps new brain cells to grow, leading to better cognitive skills.

8. **Teach Kids How Physical Activity Reduces Stress.** A brisk walk, a basketball game, or aerobics can help you relax, divert you from the causes of your stress and improve your mood and temper. If your child gets upset easily because she has a lot on her plate, get her to step back and take the time to "smell the roses" with an exercise break.

9. **Make Physical Activity a Family Event.** Simply put, by making physical activity a family event, you are not only promoting a healthy lifestyle and good family time, you are being a great role model. Place family physical activity time on your weekly calendar.

10. **Build Kids' Self-Esteem with Success.** Children with high self-esteem have confidence in their ability to perform daily tasks or face a variety of challenges in life. For some children, it is an innate quality, for others, it is acquired through life experiences. As parents, we want to build up our children's self-esteem as best we can so they have the confidence to excel in sports as well as in life. The key is to be honest, complimenting their best qualities, but at the same time keeping them grounded.

Many factors can impact a child's self-esteem. Physical appearance can be important; a child who is overweight or very tall for his age may have some insecurity that lowers self-esteem, which could hinder performance. A shy nature can bring with it difficulty communicating and a poor self-image. Cultural differences can also have a negative impact, since children frequently don't know how they should perceive cultures different from their own. Also, many children put an emphasis on material things, which can make a child whose family cannot afford "things" uncomfortable. Poor grades and a lower skill set can have a negative impact on a child's self-esteem as well. When you participate in an activity with your child, spend a little time thinking of ways for them to succeed easily for their skill level. High self-esteem can create higher skill levels through confidence-building.

A Word about Stress Management

Feeling pressured by competition isn't the only stress that can prevent your children from reaching their potential. Fear of the unknown, vulnerability, the need for approval, and personal loss can all cause stress. While small amounts of stress can be positive, because they may improve performance, teach children how to "think on their feet," and prepare them for the stress of the "real world," large amounts of stress are harmful to your child's health. Stress can affect their bodies in many ways, such as causing an increased heart rate, rapid breathing, sweating, muscle tension, and elevated blood pressure. Repeated exposure to high stress situations can produce feelings of tension and anxiety for children, even when they are involved in low or no-stress activities. The key is to reduce tension and anxiety through stress management. Here are some ways to manage your child's stress levels.

Len's Top Ten Ways to Manage Your Child's Stress and Anxiety

1. Always be aware of what is causing your child stress. Children should be encouraged to talk about what is bothering them. Think about how it's affecting them and what you can do to minimize it.

2. Take the time to smell the roses! Teach your children to slow down, take a deep breath, and relax.

3. Take some time to exercise. A nice long walk or jog can ease the mind.

4. Make sure your child gets a good night's sleep to help her focus on the task at hand.

5. Serve nutritious foods to keep your child's mind and body strong.

6. Teach your child to concentrate on one task at a time.

7. Teach your child to take frequent small breaks.

8. Take a family outing or trip, something that the entire family can enjoy doing together.

9. Plan out your child's day to avoid the stress of needing to hurry through his activities.

10. Tell your child you love her and give her plenty of positive reinforcement.

CHAPTER THREE

Getting in the Habit of Being Active

Just like smoking cigarettes or biting one's nails, leading a sedentary lifestyle is a habit that, once begun, can be very hard to break. In this chapter, we'll discuss the importance of beginning healthy habits at a young age. We'll also discuss how to break bad habits before they become hard-to-break patterns.

In my experience, kids fall into bad habits due to one or a combination of three reasons. First, bad habits are learned from a child's most important influence: you. If a child sees that you stay up late at night, spend most of your time watching television, or regularly drink caffeinated and sugary drinks, she will believe that all of these behaviors are appropriate. While it is important that a child understand that some behaviors are okay for adults but not okay for children, such as having an occasional alcoholic beverage, parents are the key to a child's understanding of which behaviors lead to a healthy lifestyle and which do not.

Second, kids may develop bad habits in an effort to seek out comfort or security. For example, when a child feels nervous, he may play with his hair, scratch himself or bite his nails. These behaviors actually cause a hormonal change which helps the body to relax, thus soothing the child when he is under stress. A child can sometimes become dependent on this response to manage all stressful situations.

Third, kids develop habits and behaviors in order to "fit in" with a group at school, such as smoking, playing video games non-stop, or just "hanging out" rather than engaging in more productive activities. This is a kind of peer pressure experienced by most kids at one time or another that often leads kids down negative paths.

It's always more difficult to break a child of a bad habit than to prevent her from forming the habit in the first place. Let's look at some tried and true ways in which you can prevent negative behaviors from becoming bad habits, then we'll look at a few ways to break a bad habit that might already have a hold on your child.

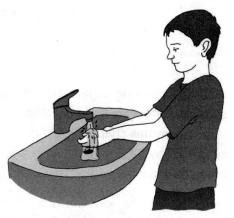

Have your children begin proper habits at a young age.

Preventing a Habit from Starting

How do you prevent a child from picking up a bad habit such as smoking, drugs, alcohol or a sedentary lifestyle? While there are no definitive answers to this question (since all situations and children are different), here are some strategies I have seen used successfully over the years.

Be a Good Role Model

When I was in college I worked at a summer camp. One camper would constantly use one particularly vulgar word in conversation and was obviously comfortable using it. As it turned out, his father used the word non-stop at home so, of course, his son thought it was fine to use it anyplace, anytime.

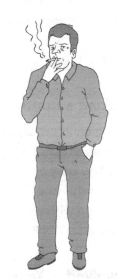

The point is that you, as the parent, must learn to live a healthy lifestyle, especially when your kids are present. Smoking, drinking, alcohol, and a sedentary lifestyle should never take place around a child. This does not mean you can't watch a television show with your child. It means that you need to lead by example. If a parent is always watching TV and never getting off the couch, a poor example is being set. Be aware that kids are watching and listening and they will emulate the behavior they see and hear at home.

Adults need to lead by example. Children tend to mimic their parents' behaviors.

Communicate at All Times

Open up lines of communication with your kids at the earliest possible age. They need to know they can always come to you and discuss what is happening in their lives no matter how painful or surprising the subject may be to you. Teaching good communication skills when your child is young will enable him to feel comfortable discussing many of the concerns he may have as he is exposed to the world. If you think your child will just start opening up to you in his teen years just because you want to monitor his life, you will be very disappointed.

Getting kids to be comfortable talking to you means you need to make a concerted effort to get involved in their lives. Ask non-invasive questions frequently, so they know you care about them; if you only ask questions when you suspect they are up to something, they may not respond to you.

Try Making a Contract with Your Child

For young children, try using a fun, non-threatening written contract between you and your child, which may assist in breaking a habit. You may be surprised at how your child responds. At the back of this book you'll find a habit-busting contract you can remove, sign with your child and display someplace (like the refrigerator door) where you'll all be sure to see it.

Get Involved in Your Child's Life

Get to know your child's friends. Sometimes, you can learn things you never knew about him through his friends, and they may give you information that might help you help your child. This works as well when you see one of your child's friends participating in some activity of which you do not approve. You can share this information with your child, who might be able to pass it along to his friends' parents.

Realize there is no magic formula when it comes to preventing habits. Watch your children closely. Notice changes in their behavior, and pay attention to questions they may ask you. Understand that all children are different. What may work with one of your children may not work with another.

Stopping a Habit

If a child does form a bad habit, how do you stop it? Here are a few methods, but you must figure out which one works best for your child. All personalities and habits are different, so all kids must be handled differently. First and foremost, try not to jump to conclusions. Kids are curious by nature, and may experiment with new things. Don't assume your child has a bad habit if he does something just one time. Consistently bad behavior, on the other hand, may need to be addressed.

Talk With the Professionals

First and foremost, if the habit is serious, seek the advice of your child's pediatrician, guidance counselor, teacher, coach, school nurse or principal. They can tell you what steps to take to help your child, which might include getting your child to end the behavior immediately ("going cold turkey") or they may suggest that the behavior be ended gradually, using positive reinforcement, which involves the use of consistent praise for your child's good behavior, more on which is discussed below. If the habit is serious enough, they may recommend medications or counseling.

Praise Works!

Praise positive behaviors! It is very important to let a child know when he does something outstanding. In general, children want to please their parents as much as they possibly can. A child is more likely to change if he knows you are viewing him positively, rather than focusing on his bad behavior. The worst thing to do is to constantly remind a child of his bad behavior, particularly in front of others. Instead of being critical, it's always a better idea to be constructive. In the same vein, never punish a bad habit.

Remember, a habit is just a coping mechanism, so try to get to the root of the problem to determine what is causing the habit.

Replace the Bad with the Good

Try not to take something away without giving something in return. For example, if you are going to take away a sugary snack, replace it with a sweet fruit. If you take away TV time from a child, replace it with a basketball or skateboard. The idea is to replace the bad behavior with a healthy, positive alternative.

Be Creative

Think about positive ways in which you can change your child's behavior. For example, if you are worried about your child eating too much at night, have him brush his teeth a little earlier in the evening so his mind is cued to believe that consuming food for the night is over.

Always Keep it Positive

Reward good behavior with something your child enjoys. For example, allow your child to play with his favorite toy or have a friend come over to the house to play.

Dealing with Peer Pressure

Peer pressure is generally understood to be persuasion by members of one's group to take a certain action, adopt certain values, or otherwise conform in order to be accepted. So, what does peer pressure have to do with bad habits? A great deal. Unfortunately, many terrible habits that young children start are a response to peer pressure. If the kids in a group are all smoking except for one child, that child may feel left out and he may start smoking in order to feel accepted. To many children, acceptance is important for social growth. As parents, we need to explain peer pressure to our kids and reinforce the positives while discouraging the negatives. Here are some exercises you can do with your children to help them cope with peer pressure.

Exercise 1—Image Imagination

Figure 3.1 illustrates peer pressure on your child. Ask her to imagine the arrows as people and explain the significance of the left arrow in the circle.

Figure 3.1

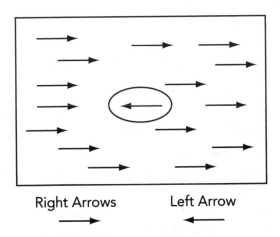

Explain that the arrows pointing to the right are children who do not exercise at all, and the arrow pointing left is a child who exercises on a daily basis. Then ask the following questions:

1. Are the right-pointing arrows correct because there are more of them?

2. What makes the left arrow so special?

3. Why is the left arrow more strong-minded than the right arrows?

4. Give an example of how she could be a left arrow.

Exercise 2—Role Play

Some nights after dinner, set up various situations with your child and have her role play how she would handle the circumstance. For example, set up a situation where a group of your child's friends are smoking cigarettes and your child comes into contact with them. It is a special group of children that your child admires, and would like to fit in with. When your child comes over, they ask her to smoke with them. How would your child handle this situation? Act out different scenarios with your child, such as: just saying no; walking away from the group; explaining the dangers of smoking; suggesting another, more healthy activity to the group.

Exercise 3—When I Was a Kid

As a child, I was always fascinated with adults and their experiences. After all, they were older and wiser, and had experienced many things I had not even heard of. Many times, what makes a new generation great is when they learn from the past mistakes of their elders. When you talk to your children, tell them about situations you had to deal with when you were a child, and how you either handled it, or should have handled it. They may learn from your experiences and be keener to listen if they understand that you once faced what they are now experiencing.

Exercise 4—Friend or No Friend

Friends are very important to a growing child. Having friends gives a child confidence, higher self-esteem, and the ability to say "no" to dangerous situations. Practice with your child different strategies for communicating with his friends the concerns he may have with the group's behavior. Teaming up with a friend against peer pressure is a great asset: it's always easier for two or more children to say "no" to a large group than it is for a child to go it alone.

Exercise 5—The Benefits and Costs of Peer Pressure

Discuss with your child both the positives and negatives of succumbing to peer pressure. He needs to think about how he might benefit, and what the costs may be of bowing to pressure, and to weigh the two together. A good exercise is set up situations for which he needs to state what the benefits and the costs are of going with the group. Examples of situations might include smoking, drinking, using drugs, stealing, bullying, skipping school, being sedentary, and dressing inappropriately.

CHAPTER FOUR

Go Offline:
Reducing Technology

Let's face it: children spend too much time using technology. I routinely poll my kids at school to find out how much time they spend each day with technology. I am always shocked to learn that the average is over four hours.

Once upon a time, most parents were not concerned about their children becoming sedentary, overweight or obese. They didn't have to be. "Playing" meant running through backyards, peddling furiously around neighborhoods and playing basketball and baseball. Move the clock ahead 30 years and a major health crisis is taking place, one aided and abetted by television, computers, video gaming, cell phones, DVDs, CDs, mp3s and mp4s, all of which are available to and adored by our children.

It's true that today's parents cannot raise their children as their parents did 30 years ago. However, while technology makes our lives easier and sometimes more exciting or fun, it is also contributing to the development of a generation of kids whose idea

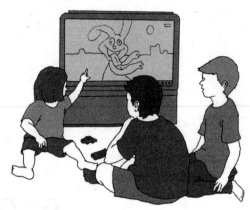

In many households, children watch between 2 and 4 hours of TV a day!

of play revolves around these cool gadgets, and a generation of busy parents who view technology as a babysitter.

In my view, technology is winning the battle for the attention and the health of our kids. If you are serious about improving your kid's health, their obsession with gadgets must be addressed. If you follow the plan I have laid out for getting kids more involved in physical activity, some of the effects of modern life will automatically be reduced. But there is more you can do. Let's look at my top ten strategies for teaching children to give up some technology while increasing their physical activity.

Len's Top Ten Strategies for Reducing Technology

1. **Institute a Technology Time Limit.** A lack of supervision and rules sometimes gives a child freedom that, once established, is hard to take away, and that freedom usually results in spending more time with technology. Simple guidelines may help to reduce this amount of sedentary time. Sit with your child and work together on a strategy that is agreeable to everyone, and then make sure everyone follows it. Figure 4.1 gives some suggestions on a strategy to reduce the time spent with technology.

Table 4.1 *Lifestyle changes over the last 30 years that have contributed to childhood obesity*

Then	Now
Most children walked to school.	Most children ride the bus.
A handful of TV stations available to kids in which many of the channels and shows were geared towards adults. The result: children lost interest in watching TV. There was no remote control; you had to get up to change a channel.	Hundreds of TV stations available to kids, including 24/7 channels designed only for children's shows that keep their attention too long. Too many remote controls to do all the work for us.
In most households, one parent worked.	In most households, both parents work.
No vending machines in schools.	Vending machines in schools.
Most children went outside to play for hours without supervision.	The majority of young children cannot go outside unless properly supervised by an adult.
Not many commercials glamorizing unhealthy food products to children.	Many commercials glamorizing unhealthy food products to children.
The cereal section at the supermarket had two shelves, with a handful of sugared cereal.	The cereal section at the supermarket has two aisles, with many sugared cereals.
Play outweighed technology.	Technology outweighs play.
Some fast foods available.	Many fast foods available.
Children communicated face to face.	Children communicate through technology.
Children went with their parents to shop, which was a great way to get some walking exercise.	Parents shop online a majority of the time.

Figure 4.1 *Strategies to Reduce Technology**

Cell phone—Limit to 3 calls per day on school days, or 20 minutes total per day.

Video games—Limit to 20 minutes per day.

Computer—Not counting homework, limit to 30 minutes per day.

Music—Limit to 20 minutes per day.

Television—Limit to 30 minutes per day.

* On weekends, you may want to extend these suggestions.

If you add up the suggested times in Figure 4.1, they equal two hours of technology time each day, an amount which is generally acceptable to most experts in child development. The suggested apportionment of time among technologies may work for some families but not others. You need to build on these suggestions to meet your family's particular needs and desires. But limits need to be set, and those limits ought to be agreed upon among you and your kids.

2. **Keep a Log of Technology Time.** Logging activity throughout the day can be a tedious job for some, but for others it is very helpful. Try it. Keep a daily log of all of the occasions your child uses the cell phone, video games, television, etc. for a full week. In many cases, this helps you and your children visualize the total amount of time they spend using technology, which will often by itself discourage them from using it so much. Obviously, the

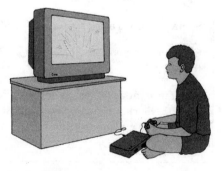

Technology does not have to be taken away completely.

intent is to get your children acclimated to a new schedule that includes much more physical activity.

3. **Make Time for Family Activities.** You are the key to a healthy child. Instead of sitting down to watch TV together, try to plan for physical activity as a family. It's a great way to reduce technology, get some exercise, and most importantly, enjoy time together as a family. Go for a walk, bike ride, play a traditional sport or walk around the mall together. Much more on this in the following chapters.

4. **Join the 2:1 Club.** The goal of the 2:1 Club is to teach children that *technology is an earned privilege, as opposed to an expected daily occurrence.* As mentioned earlier, statistics show that children watch between two and four hours of television each night. If you add other technology to this, a child may spend half his day enjoying some form of technology, with little time left for physical activity. Some type of happy medium must be found to combat this problem.

The principle behind the 2:1 Club is to make kids earn their time spent with technology through physical activity. For example, for every 2 minutes of physical activity a child engages in, they earn 1 minute of technology time. Another example would be if a child rides his bike for an hour, he gets to play video games for 30 minutes. Table 4.2 shows

Table 4.2 *The 2:1 Club: Earning Technology Time*

Time of Activity	Earned Technology Time
30 minute family walk	15 minutes
1 hour basketball game	30 minutes
20 minute bike ride	10 minutes
2 hour hike	1 hour
40 minute physical education class	20 minutes
1 hour karate class	30 minutes

different examples of how children can earn technology time by joining the 2:1 Club.

You and your child should reach an agreement about when the technology time he earns can be used. For example, if a child comes home late from karate class, he may only have time to do some homework, get a snack, shower, and get to bed; he may not have time to get his technology time in that day. In such an instance, you need to work out a plan to enable your child to "bank" his time for use another day.

Another thing to consider is the "max out" time for technology. A crafty child may manipulate his schedule to earn time that exceeds the daily limit you have placed on technology time. You may need to create a maximum amount of technology time your child can earn for each day. You might consider a two hour limit each day, whatever is consistent with the technology time limit you have set.

A formal written contract, by which your child agrees to abide by the technology rules you have set between you, motivates kids to stick with the rules. You'll find a Downtime-from-Online contract at the back of this book. Cut it out, sign it, and post it. It really works! Obviously, you can't be with your kids 24 hours a day, so the honor system does come into play: you'll have to trust your kids to follow the rules while you are not around.

5. **Try a Technology Shutdown.** How long can your family go without any modern technology? As a family, try to schedule two hours once in a while where no one uses technology. No phones, no music, no TV, no computers. See if you can survive; it might be the first time your child has gone without technology in his life. Substitute a family walk, reading, or just plain family conversation. You may be pleasantly surprised at how it turns out.

6. **Make a Schedule.** Children understand schedules very well. Many actually respond positively when they know

parts of their day are planned out for them. A good way to reduce technology is to schedule times throughout the day for family projects, which might include reading, walking, going to a park, playing board games or just talking.

7. **Make Bedrooms Technology-Free.** Throughout the years I have had the opportunity to discuss with many parents the strategies they have used to keep their kids healthy. The parents of a 5th grader once described to me their trouble keeping him away from video games and computers. From the minute he came home until he went to bed, all he wanted to do was play on the computer or with his video games. They eventually realized that the child's enthusiasm might have been affected by the fact that all of the technology was located in his bedroom, which made access way too easy for him. They found that simply moving all the equipment from their son's room, thereby automatically putting a limit on access, proved to be a successful strategy for them (although it was not their most popular decision, from their son's point of view). Be prepared, however: if you follow this strategy, your child may insist that you have no technology in your bedroom, and as a good role model, you may need to accede to your child's wishes.

8. **Limit TV Time.** Here are some suggestions to lower time with the tube:
   - Take the TV out of your child's room.
   - Schedule the times your child can watch TV.
   - Use a timer. When the timer goes off, so does the TV.
   - Record his favorite shows, and pick times acceptable to you for him to watch them.
   - Make reading time equal to TV time, not to exceed two hours. For every minute your child reads, he gets a minute of TV time.

9. **Don't Use Technology as a Babysitter.** How many of you have said to your child, at one time or another, "please

watch some TV or go on your computer" just so they would leave you alone? The point is that in some cases, parents actually encourage their child to use too much technology. Try to be aware of the number of times you point your child to the television. Remember: once begun, bad habits are hard to break.

10. **Don't Ban Technology Completely.** It's never a good idea to shut your kids off completely from technology. This will cause resentment and may affect the way they interact with other kids. Simply reducing, not ending, a kid's relationship with technology is the better course to follow.

Let's pause for a moment to review Part I of this book. We've discussed the problems associated with childhood inactivity and given you the tools to determine the work you and your children will need to do to ensure their health now and for the future. We've looked at how children view the world of competition and given you ways to approach your own children's possible aversion to exercise. You've learned proven methods for managing the stress and anxiety that may be negatively impacting your kids. What's more, we've spelled out proven methods for turning their bad habits into good ones: good habits that can include healthy activity a positive attitude towards their own health.

Now it's time to put all this information into action and start reaping the rewards. Let's go!

PART TWO

The Action Plan for Keeping Kids Fit

CHAPTER FIVE

Get Moving:
The Benefits of Exercise

Most credible health organizations suggest that children need approximately 60 minutes of physical activity each day to stay healthy. While most young children cannot and should not do adult-style workouts because their endurance levels are not yet fully developed, any type of safe physical activity at any time throughout the day is acceptable, including controlled hobbies such as karate, swim club, recreation teams and organized sports. The activity need not be continuous, rather, it can be broken up into various events throughout the day, as long as the amount of time being active totals one hour.

There are five different types of exercise, defined by their effect on the body. They include cardiovascular endurance, muscle strength, muscle endurance, body composition, and flexibility. In the next few pages we'll take a closer look at each, and at how your child can excel in each area. Remember, what works for one child may not work for another, so be sure to choose appropriate exercises for your kids. And be consistent! Your children won't show any benefits if they don't exercise on a regular basis.

Cardiovascular Endurance

Cardiovascular endurance is the most important aspect of fitness. It is a measure of how strong your heart is. High cardiovascular endurance can potentially add years to one's life. It is improved and maintained by *aerobic exercise*. Aerobic means "with oxygen," and refers to an exercise using oxygen as the prime source of energy for the exercise. It requires one to breathe in more air for a longer duration while using the larger muscle groups, such as the muscles of the legs. A bike ride, a walk, or a jog for 20 to 30 minutes is considered aerobic exercise, as long as one maintains a steady pace and an elevated heart rate without a rest. Other examples of aerobic exercise include jumping rope, swimming,

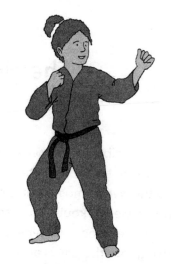

Children need approximately 60 minutes per day of physical activity.

kick boxing, inline skating or rollerblading, rowing, cross country skiing and aerobic dance. Some of the many benefits of aerobic exercise include:

1. Making the body more efficient at delivering oxygen throughout the body by increasing the number of red blood cells which carry oxygen.
2. Improving the strength of the heart.
3. Burning excess calories so they will not be stored as fat, aiding in weight control.

4. Lowering the risk factors for heart disease.
5. Lowering cholesterol.
6. Enhancing cognitive skills.
7. Lowering the chance of contracting type 2 diabetes.
8. Making the muscles stronger.
9. Increasing bone strength.
10. Increasing body metabolism.

Aerobic exercise is a great way to burn calories. For example, an individual may burn 10 calories per minute while performing a slow jog, so jogging for 20 minutes could burn off approximately 200 calories. Keep in mind that there are many factors that must be considered in determining the amount of calories burned during any exercise. For example, an individual may burn more calories by running faster, since there is more effort involved in the task. An individual who is overweight may burn more calories due to the amount of extra effort needed to perform a task. A person who has more lean body mass as opposed to fat body mass may shed more calories, because his or her body knows how to effectively burn the calories during exertion. Moreover, a body that is properly hydrated can more efficiently burn off fat as energy during a workout, which may also affect the number of calories burned.

Muscle Strength

Muscle strength, the ability of our muscles to resist greater loads, is enhanced by performing *anaerobic exercise*. Anaerobic activity requires short bursts of energy without using oxygen as the energy source of that activity. Rather, glycogen, a form of starch stored in the liver and muscles, is used as energy during anaerobic exercise. Glycogen is produced when our bodies break down carbohydrates in the food that we eat into glucose. (We'll hear more about glycogen later.) Muscular strength workouts require a short duration of high intensity exercise, such as weight lifting.

The benefits of muscular strength exercises include increased muscle mass, increased lean body mass and decreased body fat, improved metabolism, a strengthening of the tendons, joints and ligaments, an increase in bone density, improved coordination, greater heart strength, improved cholesterol levels and improved sleeping patterns. Examples of light strength training exercises that are appropriate for children include curling, bench pressing, pull-ups, curl-ups, abdominal crunches, lunges and squats. Strength training formats that include power lifting, circuit training, station training, and compound exercises are usually not recommended for younger children, but may begin under proper supervision with children in their later teens.

Whether children should participate in strength training exercise has been hotly debated over the years, but it's evident that when strength training is performed correctly, children can benefit with higher self esteem, better injury protection and recovery and increased motor performance. Keep in mind that strength training for children is safe, *only* when properly performed and supervised.

A child must use the proper "resistance," or the proper amount of weight so that he performs the number of repetitions of the exercise needed to increase muscle strength without risking injury. A child should be able to safely lift the weight 12 to 15 times in a row. If a child is only able to lift a weight 4 to 8 times in a row, too much weight is being used. Kids should concentrate on the larger muscle groups when they strength train, such as the muscles of the legs and back. As a child progresses and is able to lift the weight more than 15 times in a row, the weight should be increased by 1 to 2 pounds at a time until the child has adapted to this new weight. Children should not strength train every day, but at most every other day, to ensure that the muscles have had sufficient time to rest and recover, thereby avoiding injury. Proper breathing techniques are also important: the child should exhale from the mouth when performing the work, while breathing in through the nose during the opposing range of motion.

The general rule of thumb for strength training for younger children is to keep it simple, and that you understand the following principles of weight training.

The Overload Principle

Power should be gradually increased in order to cause adaptation, that is, when repeating an activity or skill, the body is able to adapt to the stress, and the activity becomes easier to perform. Factors that can be used to overload a muscle include load (the amount of weight used), volume (the number of repetitions of a single exercise), rest, duration (the amount of time spent exercising), and frequency (the number of workouts performed in a given period of time). Once the body has adapted to an exercise regimen, one or more of these factors need to be manipulated to yield continuing progress.

Progression

Progression is a gradual increase in the intensity of the exercise. To avoid injury, the amount of weight used and the duration of the exercises should be increased slowly. On the other hand, increasing the intensity of the workout too slowly may not yield any appreciable increase in strength.

Specificity of Training

This means working out a specific muscle to increase the strength of that muscle. The exercise must be specific to the type of strength required to improve a particular skill. For example, someone who is going to run a marathon will train by running long distances. A skier will train by skiing or performing exercises that assist with skiing. A baseball pitcher may throw a medicine ball to increase his throwing strength.

Rest and Recovery

Muscles need sufficient time to recover from the stress of training, so it's necessary to strength train different muscle groups every other day.

Muscle Endurance

While muscle strength requires short bursts of energy through the use of heavier weight and fewer repetitions of an exercise, muscle endurance, the ability of muscles to work over a longer period of time, refers to a mixture of strength and endurance. Oxygen, instead of glycogen, is used as an energy source during endurance exercises.

Muscular endurance activities are safer for children than muscle strength exercises and make the muscles stronger without bulking them up, as occurs with strength exercise. They can help a child learn proper body mechanics (the way the body moves and avoids injury), balance, rhythm, and flexibility to better prepare him for muscular strength exercises. I strongly recommended them for pre-teens. The benefits of muscle endurance exercises are the same as for muscle strength exercises with the additional benefits of flexibility, balance and rhythm. Some examples of muscle endurance exercise include distance running, weight training (low intensity, high repetition), pushups, sit-ups and curl-ups, jumping rope, raking leaves, vacuuming, swimming, bike riding, mountain climbing and hiking.

A child's physical condition determines how much and how often this type of exercise should be performed. Kids should choose an activity that is challenging but that will not overwork their muscles. Here's an example of an appropriate exercise for kids. On a chosen day, say Sunday, have your child perform as many pushups as she can until she fatigues. Let's assume your child completed 60 pushups before stopping. A good foundation for training would then be 3 sets of pushups using 50% of their maximum number every Sunday, Tuesday, and Thursday (Figure 5.1).

Figure 5.1 *Pushups Example*

Maximum performed—60 pushups

50% of maximum—30 pushups

Using this formula, the child should do 3 sets of 30 pushups every other day. When she is able to complete this regimen easily, it's time for a change. Increase the number of pushups to 75% of the maximum (Figure 5.2).

Figure 5.2 *Pushups Example*

Maximum performed—60 pushups

75% of maximum—45 pushups

Using this formula, the child should do 3 sets of 45 pushups every other day.

When this becomes too easy, it's time to test your child again for the maximum number of pushups and change the formula as appropriate. Of course, the maximum number should have risen higher than the previous testing day for the regimen to change. This process can be followed with other exercises as well. For timed events, such as walking or jogging, set a time goal for your child to achieve. For example, have your child walk a mile and set a 15-minute time limit to complete the exercise. Once that becomes too easy, reduce the time to 14 minutes, and keep reducing the time until your child can walk a 12-minute mile. Then increase the distance your child will walk, and start the process again.

Body Composition

Body composition is the ratio of body fat to lean body mass. Basic exercise, along with proper nutrition, sleep, and hydration, contribute to increasing lean body mass. While there are many ways to measure a child's body composition, the most common is the use of a child's BMI (Body Mass Index). The BMI is a number, derived from height and weight measurements, that gives a general indication of whether your weight falls within a healthy range. Although there are many online charts, graphs, and percentiles of what a child's BMI should be, I strongly recommend a visit to your child's pediatrician to get an accurate report of your child's body mass index. There is less room for error, the doctor will be able to tell you if your child fits into a healthy range and the doctor can give you specific recommendations on improving your child's health.

Body mass is not the same as body weight, but many parents use a child's weight as a measure of good health. In many cases this is inaccurate. For example, lean body mass weighs more than fat mass, which will indicate a higher weight in a child. If a child hydrates his body properly, this may also increase body weight. For these reasons, parents should have their child's pediatrician take a BMI with each routine visit.

Flexibility

Flexibility is the ability of the body to stretch to prevent injury and improve performance. Think of a pencil versus a rubber band. When a pencil bends, it breaks. A rubber band can bend and stretch, making its performance stronger and more durable. Thus, a lack of flexibility leads to poor performance and possible injury. Children easily understand this concept.

Some of the many benefits of flexibility exercises include improved range of motion, injury prevention, faster and easier acclimation to various movements and exercises, the use of less energy to perform a given task, a reduction in muscle soreness, increased blood flow to the muscles, and improved coordination. Examples of flexibility training include:

1. **Dynamic stretching.** When the individual uses the force of a muscle and the body's momentum to take a joint through the full range of motion. For example, a baseball pitcher may move his arms forward as a swimmer would perform the butterfly stroke, or a soccer player kicking an imaginary ball forward then back.

2. **Static active stretching.** The holding and maintaining of extended positions while using only the muscles. An example of this is a child lying on her back keeping one leg flat on the ground while the other leg is at a 90-degree angle.

3. **Static passive stretching.** The ability to hold a stretch using body weight or other external means. For example, doing the leg stretch described above, but with a friend holding the foot in the 90-degree angle position. In this case, the individual's muscles are passively taken to a point of tension and held there by external means.

Okay, now you understand the components of fitness, which will help you teach your children about healthy lifestyles and making wise choices. Now let's look at some ways to use this information to benefit your kids. There is no one right way to keep kids fit, and you can choose to take up some of the following suggestions, or make up your own, following the guidelines I have laid out for you. Be sure to mix up the routine you use to keep it fresh for your child.

CHAPTER SIX

First Things First: Warm-Ups and Stretching

You may already be exercising with your kids, or you may just be starting out. In either case, it's very important to make sure your kids limber up every day before exercising (and that goes for you, too). This will make the routine less likely to cause aches and pains, and will make it more enjoyable as well. You and your kids need not perform every one of these warm-ups before you exercise, but you should all agree on a few before you start.

Len's Top Ten Warm-Up and Stretch Exercises

1. **Toe Touches**
    Sitting on your bottom, point your toes straight up in the air. Keep your legs straight. Take a deep breath, and slowly bend at the hips and bring your fingers toward your toes. Reach as far as you can without rocking or rounding your spine, and hold the stretch for 5 to 10 seconds. After you've held the stretch, relax back to the starting position and repeat this 5 times.

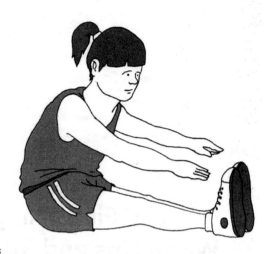

Toe touches

2. "V" Sit

Similar to the stretch above, but extend your feet and legs into the letter 'V.' Stretch forward and hold your hands directly between your legs for 5 to 10 seconds. Repeat this stretch 5 times. Next, reach both hands toward your right foot, and hold the stretch for 5 to 10 seconds. After 5 repetitions, repeat the process with the left foot.

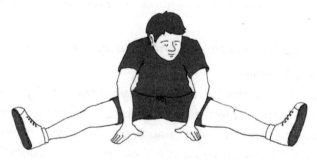

"V" sit

3. Butterfly Stretch

Sitting in the upright position with your knees bent and the soles of your feet together, place both hands on the top part of your ankles, so that your thumbs face in towards each other. Slowly bring your upper body down towards

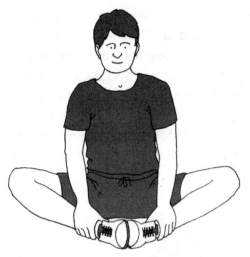

Butterfly stretch

your feet as far as you can without rocking, and hold the stretch for 5 to 10 seconds. Repeat this process 5 times.

4. Arm Circles

Stand up straight with your feet shoulder width apart. Bring both arms up so they are perpendicular with your legs (your body should look like a lower-case

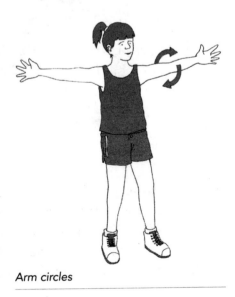

Arm circles

letter 't'). Rotate your arms in small circles 10 times forward and then 10 times backward. After you complete this exercise, rest, and perform again making medium-sized circles and then large circles.

5. Lunge Stretch

Place both hands on the ground shoulder width apart with your head tilted up. Extend one leg backwards, keeping the leg straight. Keep the other leg bent forward, with the foot flat on the ground and the knee between the hands. Lean forward slowly, making sure the front foot remains flat on the ground. Do not let the bent knee extend past the toes of the front foot. Don't let the back leg bend. Hold for 5 to 10 seconds and then switch the positions of the legs. Repeat 5 times for each leg.

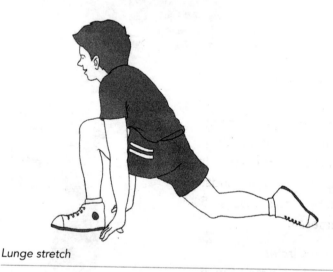

Lunge stretch

6. Four Stretches

Sit on your bottom with your right leg straight, toes pointed up. The left leg is bent with the knee facing outwards, and the sole of the foot resting against the inner thigh of the straight leg. Bring your head down towards the

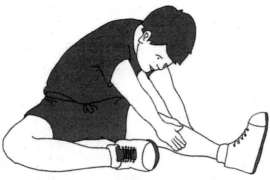

Four stretches

knee of the straight leg, and hold the stretch for 5 to 10 seconds without bouncing. After 5 to 10 seconds, relax, and rotate the positions of the legs so the left leg is now straight and the right leg is bent. Bring your head down towards the straight leg and hold the stretch for 5 to 10 seconds. Repeat the stretch 5 times.

7. Side Bends

Stand up straight with your feet shoulder width apart. Place your right hand on your hip and your left arm over your head. Bend to the right so your left hand starts going down towards your right hip. Hold that stretch for 5 to 10 seconds, then relax and switch the positions of your hands to repeat the process on the other side of your body. Repeat this stretch 5 times.

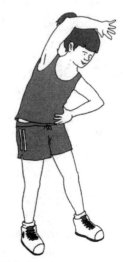

Side bends

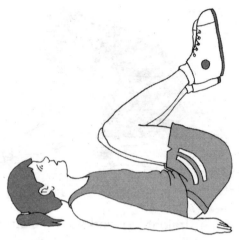

Lower back stretch

8. **Lower Back Stretch**

   Lying on your back, with the arms at the sides, bring both knees up to the chest and hug the knees in close to your body. Hold for 5 to 10 seconds. Relax back to the starting position and repeat the stretch 5 times.

9. **Calf Stretch**

   Stand up straight approximately 1 foot away from a wall. Place both hands flat on the wall, making sure your feet are shoulder width apart. Staying flat on your feet, with knees slightly bent, lean towards the wall until you feel some force on your calf muscles. Hold the stretch for 5 to 10 seconds, relax, and repeat the stretch 5 times.

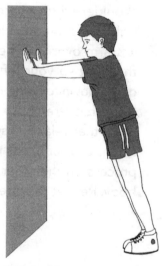

Calf stretch

10. Picking Apples

Stand up straight with the legs shoulder width apart. Reach up towards the
sky with your right hand as high as you
can, as you would pick an apple from a
tree. While you bring the right hand
down, start lifting the left hand up as
high as you can to pick more apples.
Continue this process for 20 seconds,
rest, and try it again.

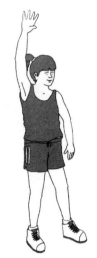

Picking apples

CHAPTER SEVEN

A Week of Family Fitness and Fun

Okay, you have learned the basic theories behind exercise, and you and your kids have warmed up and are ready to begin. In this chapter, I've set out a week's worth of fitness programs that everyone in the family can enjoy together. You don't have to follow these activities as they are set out; you can enjoy them in any order that fits your needs. You need not even follow each of them; you can make up your own. However, remember that all kids should get at least one hour of physical activity under their belts every day. Whatever you decide to do, do something every day.

Sunday is for Calisthenics

Calisthenics is a great activity for Sunday. For several of the exercises listed below, you can use the formula mentioned in Chapter 5 (Figures 5.1 and 5.2) to decide how many repetitions your child should perform in each set. It's likely that all of the exercises listed below will be far too many for your child to complete in one day. One option is to split up the exercises and perform them over a 2 to 3 day period. In many of the examples your child's body weight is used as the resistance, so very little equipment will be needed.

1. Pushups

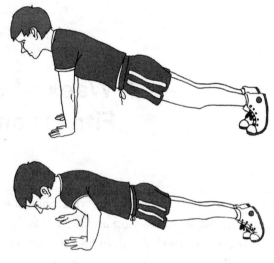

Pushups

The child starts in the elevated pushup position (top). The body must be perfectly straight, head facing forward. The child proceeds to lower to the down position by bending at the elbows (bottom). Once the chest touches the ground, and without resting on the ground, the child pushes back up to the starting position. He should not bounce off the floor in an effort to gain momentum back to the up position. The knees should not touch the ground. Allow rest at any time. Pushups are a great way to strengthen the bicep and tricep muscles of the arms, as well as the larger pectoral muscles of the chest. Have him try 3 sets of this exercise, with a sufficient rest in between sets.

2. **Curl-ups/Sit-ups**

Curl-ups strengthen the abdominal muscles in the stomach area. A curl-up is an exercise from the sit-up family, and I recommend that children do curl-ups, as they put less pressure on the spine and neck than do sit-ups. The child starts

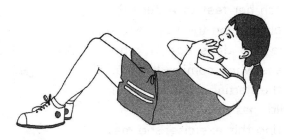

Curl-ups/Sit-ups

by lying on the floor, knees bent and arms crossed in front. The child rises up and forward until her chest touches her raised knees. Once this occurs, she must then go back to the starting position. A partner may hold the child's feet in place on the floor. Rest at any time as needed. It is recommended that a child do this exercise on a soft surface, such as a foam mat. Once again, use the formula in Chapter 5 to determine how many curl-ups to do. Your child should execute 3 sets with adequate rest in between sets.

3. **Squats**

Have the child stand up straight with her legs about shoulder width apart and her ankles, knees and hips in a straight line. Make sure her arms are raised directly in front during the entire exercise so the arms form a 90-degree angle with the legs. Start by having the child bend at the knees and lower the body as if she were going to sit on a chair until the child's buttock is in a straight line with her knees, making sure the back remains straight during the movement. If the child cannot go down that far, have her do the best she can. Have her hold the sitting position for 2 seconds, and then slowly rise back up to the starting position. The child should be pushing up through the heels, so watch her feet to ensure the heels stay on the floor. Make sure she does not lock her knees when coming back up to the starting position. If your child has trouble balancing during this exercise, she may

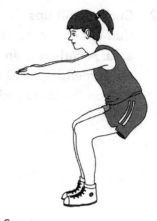

Squats

use a wall to place her hands on for support, or place a chair in front of her if she feels like she may fall backwards. Squats will help strengthen your child's abdominal muscles, quadriceps, the hamstring muscles of the legs, the gluteus muscles and the back.

Try having your child perform 10 squats at a slow and steady pace, without rushing. Once she gets to 10, allow sufficient rest, and then repeat the process two more times. If 10 squats become too easy, increase the number of squats to 11, 12, or even 15 in each set.

4. **Chin-ups/Pull-ups**

The child starts by hanging by the hands on the bar with arms fully extended, feet off the ground. A chin-up (left) has the palms of the hands facing in, while a pull-up (right) has the palms facing out. The child must pull himself up until the chin is slightly above the bar. Once this is accomplished, he must then go back down to the starting position. He may not push off any walls, nor swing his legs or arms in an effort to build momentum. For safety, the child may stop at any time by standing on the floor below the

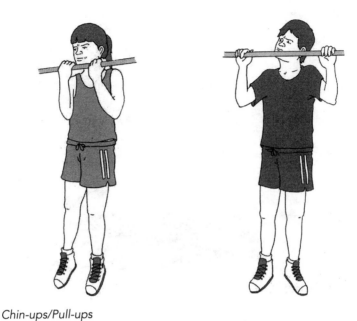

Chin-ups/Pull-ups

bar. These exercises are a great way to strengthen the bicep and tricep muscles, as well as the larger muscles of the neck and upper and mid-back. For most children, a chin-up is a little easier to perform than a pull-up. Pull-ups and chin-ups use the full weight of the body as resistance, which can cause many children to struggle during these exercises. Start them off performing these exercises one time, until they get the hang of it.

5. **Leg Raises**
Lying on his back with legs straight up in the air forming a 90-degree angle, have the child lower his legs downward, stopping a couple of inches above the ground, while keeping his back flat on the floor. Once this is completed, the legs are returned to the starting position. This exercise will strengthen your child's abdominal muscles. A variation of this exercise is the single leg raise. The child sets up for the exercise the same way as with the double leg raise. Keeping his back flat on the floor, the child lowers the right leg

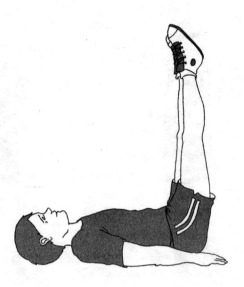

Leg Raises

down to just above to the ground, then steadily brings it back up to meet the left leg. The child alternates between right and left legs for the desired number of repetitions.

Have your child try this exercise 10 times. Once completed, give him a rest period, and repeat the process two more times. When 10 repetitions become too easy, increase to 11, 12, or even 15 repetitions per set, and keep increasing by 1 leg raise each time the exercise becomes too easy. When doing single leg raises, one "rep" equals lowering and raising both the right and left leg.

6. **Jumping Jacks**
Starting off in a standing position with the feet together and arms at the sides, jump in the air and separate the feet. As the feet separate, the arms are brought up above the head. Once the hands are in the "up" position, jump the feet together again, bringing the arms back down to the starting position. Jumping jacks use a variety of muscles throughout the body including the hamstrings, quadri-

ceps, and gastrocnemius muscles in the legs, the abdominal muscles and the biceps and triceps muscles.

Some younger children will find the body mechanics and timing of jumping jacks challenging, and may get frustrated trying to complete several jumping jacks in a row. If your child has a difficult time coordinating his upper and lower body during a full jumping jack, you can break the exercise down for him. First have him stand with feet together and arms by his sides.

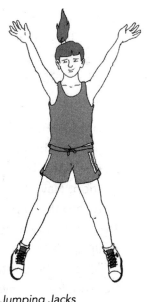

Jumping Jacks

Without jumping or moving his legs, have the child bring his arms and hands away from the body and up in the air, and continue to bring the arms back down to the starting position. Have him practice this movement several times until he is comfortable with it.

Next, have your child stand in the starting position and keep the hands and arms steady by his sides. From here, the child will jump his feet apart and then quickly back together. He should practice this jumping movement until he is comfortable and can do up to 15 "leg jacks" in a row. When your child can complete both the upper and lower segments of jumping jacks individually, he is ready to combine the two for a full jumping jack. You will want to have him begin slowly, in order for him to get the timing and rhythm correct for a full jumping jack.

Some kids can complete hundreds of jumping jacks without tiring out. Pick a number for him to start off this exercise, and have him execute 3 sets of the number chosen. For example, start off with 25 jumping jacks per set. When that becomes too easy, increase it by increments of 5 until he reaches 100. If jumping jacks start to become too easy, try a more challenging skill, like jumping rope.

7. **Shoulder Rolls**
   Your child should place her arms at her side while standing at attention. Have her lift her shoulders into the "up" position, and then roll them forward while pulling them in slightly. She child should continue moving her shoulders forward in a circular motion until they have rotated 360 degrees. This exercise helps strengthen the trapezius and deltoid muscles in the upper back and neck. Have your child try this exercise 10 times, and then repeat it in a backward movement 10 more times. Performing 3 sets of this exercise in both directions is a good warm-up.

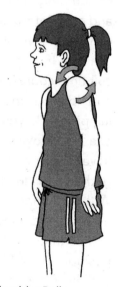

Shoulder Rolls

8. **Lunges**
   Lunges are a great way to work on the leg muscles, and assist with balance and coordination. Standing up straight with the legs about shoulder width apart, hands at the sides, have your child step forward with one leg, bending at the knee to lower his body. He does not need to step very far, and must keep his back straight. Make sure your his front knee does not extend past his foot as he bends, and to keep the front foot perpendicular to the floor.

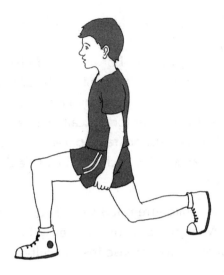

Lunges

Move back to the starting position and repeat with the other leg. This exercise works the buttocks, quadriceps, hamstrings, and calf muscles of the legs. Try having your child perform 3 sets of 10 alternating lunges at a slow and steady pace, without rushing. He should lunge forward with the left leg, come back to the starting position, and then lunge forward with the right leg, and come back to the starting position.

9. **Calf Raises**

Have your child stand on the floor with his feet pointing forward and about one foot apart. Keeping the knees straight but not locked tightly in place, he then raises himself up to the balls of the feet and squeezes

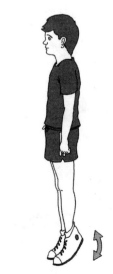

Calf Raises

the calves, moving only at the ankles. He should remain in the "up" position for a second, and then release back to the starting position. For an added challenge, have your child stand on a phone book, curb, or step with his heels hanging off the back. Have him follow the same directions. This exercise is great for the calf muscles. If you do use the phone book, curb, or stairs, parental supervision is necessary to make sure your child is in a safe area and does not fall down.

Have your child attempt 3 sets of 10 repetitions of this exercise. When this becomes too easy, have him use a book, curb, or stairs to increase the difficulty.

10. Chair Dips

Have your child sit in a chair with her hands placed firmly on the arms and her legs extended straight ahead resting on the heels of her feet. Be sure she does not lock her legs too tightly. She should lift her buttocks off the front of the chair until both arms are fully extended, and then bend the elbows and lower her body down until the elbows are at a

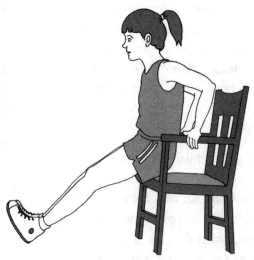

Chair Dips

90-degree angle. Do not allow the buttocks to touch the seat. Push up and repeat the exercise. This is a great exercise for the triceps and pectoral muscles. As with pull-ups and chin-ups, dips use a great deal of the child's body weight for resistance. I recommend that your child practice this exercise with supervision until she gets the hang of it. Have her work up to sets of 5, and as she gets stronger, sets of 10.

11. Crisscross

Have your child lie on his back, with the shoulders 3 to 5 inches off the ground and the heels raised up off the floor. The mid and lower sections of the back should remain pressed to the floor while the abdominal muscles are kept tight. The arms are at the sides on the floor. The exercise

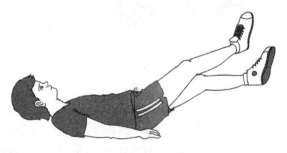

Crisscross

starts by crossing the left foot over the top of the right foot. Without stopping, rotate the feet so the right foot now crosses over the left. Without resting, continue this alternating pattern. This exercise will strengthen your child's abdominal muscles. Try having your child perform 10 alternating crisscrosses at a slow and steady pace, without rushing. Give him sufficient rest, and have him try it two more times.

12. Scissors

The set up for this exercise is the same as for the crisscross. Start by raising the legs up approximately 5 inches, and back down to the starting position, while keeping the legs straight. The movement of the legs should be completed in an alternating motion; this means while the right leg is moving up, the left leg is moving down. Once this is complete, the legs rotate as the left leg starts to move up, and the right leg comes down. This exercise will strengthen your child's abdominal muscles.

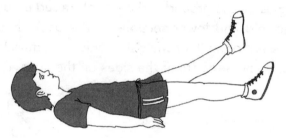

Scissors

For a change, try making this a timed activity. For example, have your child try to do this exercise continuously for 10 seconds, rest, and repeat the cycle two more times. If you find that 10 seconds is too easy, increase the time to make it challenging.

13. Leg Crab Kicks

Have your child get into the crab walk position: lying on her back, she lifts the buttocks in the air while supporting herself with the hands and feet. Once in the crab walk position, she should kick out the right leg in the air, leaving the body supported by both hands and the left leg. Bring the right leg back to the starting position, and repeat the process with the left leg now coming up in the air. This exercise will strengthen your child's abdominal muscles, bi-

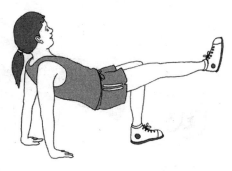

Leg Crab Kicks

ceps, and triceps. As with the scissors exercise, make this a timed activity. Have her try for 10 seconds, rest, and repeat the cycle two more times. If 10 seconds is too easy, increase the time to make it challenging.

14. No Rope Jump Rope

In a standing position, have your child start jumping up and down, creating a comfortable rhythm while moving the arms in a circular motion. She will be strengthening many muscles in the lower and upper body. This exercise can also be timed. Have her try to do this for 20 seconds, rest, and repeat the cycle two more times. Again, increase the time if this becomes too easy.

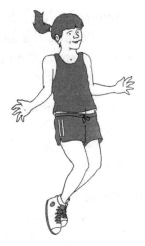

No Rope Jump Rope

15. Chest Touch Pushups

This exercise starts in the elevated pushup position, keeping the body perfectly straight, with the crown of the head facing forward. The child lowers himself to the down position by bending at the elbows. Once the chest touches the ground and without resting on the ground, he then pro-

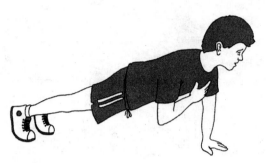

Chest Touch Pushups

ceeds back up to the starting position. As he gets close to the starting position, he must bring his right hand up towards the left part of the chest so both feet and the left hand support the body. Once completed, the right hand is brought back down to the ground and he then lowers himself back to the pushup position. On the way up, he now brings the left hand up towards the right part of the chest and follows the same pattern. Chest pushups are a great way to strengthen the bicep and tricep muscles of the arms and the pectoral muscles of the chest.

Use the formula found in Chapter 5 (Figure 5.1) to decide how many chest pushups your child should perform. Once that is calculated, have him try three sets of this exercise, with a sufficient rest in between sets.

16. Prone Plank

Have your child lie face down, resting on the forearms with feet together. Push the floor away to separate the shoulder

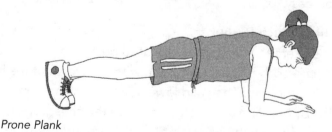

Prone Plank

blades and tuck the chin, creating a straight line from the top of head to the heels. Keep the body in straight alignment, with arms parallel to the body. This exercise will help to develop your child's core strength, which will aid in good posture and better-developed abdominal muscles.

The child should perform this exercise in a timed format. You can begin with 15 seconds, and work up to holding the prone plank for 30 seconds. The ultimate goal will be to hold the plank for 60 seconds.

17. Mountain Climbers

Have your child set up in pushup position with a straight alignment of the spine. The child will then lift one leg and pull it into the chest without rounding the spine, holding the knee in for 2 seconds and then returning to the starting position. Have your child alternate legs, as if he were climbing up a mountain.

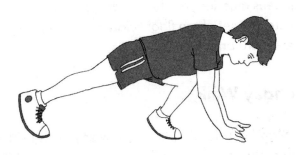

Mountain Climbers

Begin with 5 repetitions. Remember that one repetition is completed when both the right and then the left knee come up into the chest. Work up to one set of 10 repetitions, and eventually two to three sets of 10 repetitions.

18. Two-leg Floor Bridge

Have your child lie down on his back with knees bent, feet flat on the floor, hip-distance apart. The arms should be at the child's side, resting on the floor, palms down. Have your

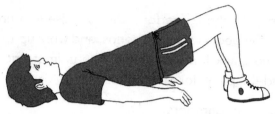

Two-leg Floor Bridge

child draw his belly button in, and push through the heels of both feet to lift the hips and pelvis off the floor. The knees, hips, and shoulders should now be in a straight line. Have your child slowly lower the hips and pelvis back to the floor. The floor bridge is a great exercise to activate the gluteus muscles and the quadriceps. Have your child complete one set of ten floor bridges. In time, work up to three sets of 10 bridges.

A Monday Walk

Make Monday a family walk day. Many people don't realize walking is the most comprehensive exercise, and it can easily get overlooked by many families. In fact, the simple act of walking has an amazing list of benefits. For most people, it has a high degree of success and does not require athletic ability. It's also a great family activity that all ages can do together, with no competition, equipment, or risk of injury. Walking relaxes the body and stimulates the heart and blood flow, which enhance cognitive skills. It can help reduce the risk of many illnesses, such as heart disease and type 2 diabetes, and strengthens the im-

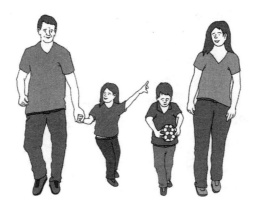

mune system. A good walk can also help keep you energized and focused during the day while helping you fall asleep at night.

Encourage your children to walk with you for 30 to 40 minutes without taking a rest while maintaining a steady pace for the entire walk. Walking is great for increasing muscle endurance, and walking for long periods at a fast pace can also be a fun aerobic activity. To increase flexibility and reduce stress, do a short stretch/warm-up before and after the walk, as described in Chapter 6.

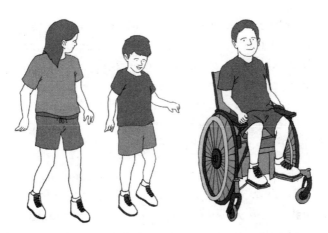

Walking is a great source of exercise, easy to perform anywhere.

How to Walk Correctly

We walk every day, but many children do not do it correctly. This may take a toll on the body, over time. Many adults today have serious issues with various joints, poor posture, or even their spine due to walking incorrectly for so many years. Parents need to focus on walking correctly so their children will literally follow in their footsteps.

Basic Walking Tips

- Get a medical checkup before starting a walking program.

- Pick a safe location for your children to walk, keeping away from busy roads and intersections. If you walk at night, make sure your children are wearing reflectors or light colors.

- Avoid wearing headphones while walking so you can pay attention to the surrounding area and the safety of your children.

- Pick comfortable sneakers to walk in. Using flip-flops, sandals, or non-athletic shoes to walk in can be very damaging over a period of time.

- Use your arms when you walk. Many children leave them dangling at the sides, but they should actually move back and forth when in travel. They can come up as high as a 90-degree angle when a child is walking faster. When the left leg is forward, the right arm should be forward and vice versa. This helps balance the body, maintain good posture, and distribute the weight evenly.

- Know when to slow your child's pace, especially if she cannot carry on a conversation normally (gasping for air) while in travel. If the walking is too easy for your child, there is nothing wrong with picking up the pace a little to get the heart rate up.

- Try at least 30 minutes of walking each night. Many health experts say it is okay to break it up into 3-ten minute intervals if you cannot do 30 continuous minutes.

- Try not to let your children walk on their toes. Their feet should roll from the heel to toe, pushing off their toes as they move forward.

- Feet should be pointed straight forward, not inverted or everted. If your child experiences pain when the toes point straight out, talk with your pediatrician.

- Teach your children to walk without hunching their backs or with their heads slumped forward. This is a common problem associated with poor sleeping habits, as children do not have the strength or stamina to maintain their good posture. It is important for children to get plenty of sleep to allow them to focus on the proper mechanics of walking.

- Teach your children to stretch before they walk to prevent injury.

- Have your children pick a natural, comfortable stride when walking. Some children take too short a stride, which may put too much pressure on their heels, while others take too long a stride, which may be hard on their joints and bad for their coordination while walking.

Don't Forget to Cool Down

When your family finishes its walk for the day, spend a few minutes doing a cool down to reduce stress on your muscles, including your heart. Cooling down helps your heart rate and breathing to return to normal gradually, which is less stressful on the body. Try to walk at a slower pace at the end of your walk, followed by some easy stretching. This will also help reduce the chances of cramps or lightheadedness. A gradual slowdown allows you to sweat, which is the body's mechanism for cooling you off after exercise.

Len's Top Ten Walking Activities

1. **10,000 Steps.** Many health professionals believe taking 10,000 steps a day is a great walking activity. Many children may find it fun to wear a pedometer (a device that measures how many steps you take for an extended period of time) to see how many steps they are taking throughout the day. They do not need to take 10,000 steps, but have them set realistic goals for themselves, and then have them try to beat their own personal best. You can find inexpensive pedomoeters at many sporting good stores.

2. **Family Walks.** Walking as a family promotes family time, conversation, and exercise. Make it a daily activity throughout the year.

3. **Walking Dogs.** Take your dog or the neighbor's dog for a long relaxing walk as a great exercise session.

4. **Tree, 1, 2, and 3.** Go to your local park with your family. On "go," walk around the park in a safe area, and see how many different trees you can touch in 2 minutes.

5. **Use the Stairs.** Instead of taking the elevator or escalator, use the stairs the get the blood flowing.

6. **Walk a Mile.** Go to your local high school track and see if your family can walk around the track 4 times, which equals one mile.

7. **Walk to School.** If you live close enough to your school and the weather is cooperative, try walking instead of driving the car or riding the bus.

8. **Mall Shop.** The mall is a great place to walk.

9. **Walking Baseball.** Find a local baseball field, and try walking the bases a designated amount of times.

10. **Color Walk.** Go to your local park, pick a color, and everyone must walk to that color. Once complete, pick a new color, then everyone must walk to the new color.

Tuesday is Household Chores Day

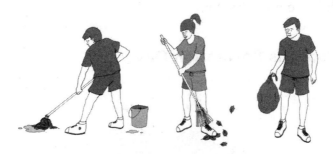

Household chores prevent children from being sedentary.

Doing household chores not only teaches children about responsibility and making a contribution to their family, but can also be exercise. Simple chores like taking out the garbage, vacuuming, raking leaves, painting, mopping the floor and shoveling the snow can all keep children fit.

Sports on Wednesday

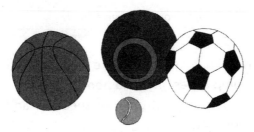

Pick a day during your week to be sports day.

Sports are a great way to promote family interaction and are also a fun way to get some exercise. Pick a couple of sports to play that the children enjoy, such as soccer, kickball, basketball, or tennis. These sports will allow your child to develop hand-eye (and hand-foot) coordination while participating in an aerobic exercise. Sports also help children understand the nature of rules and help build character as they learn good sportsmanship. We'll discuss the role of sports in your child's life in greater depth in the next chapter.

Thursday is Recreation Day

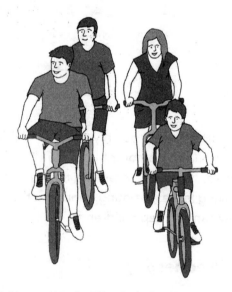

Recreational activities can involve the whole family.

Take a family swim, bike ride, or hike to get your daily exercise. Pull out the jump ropes and hula hoops for a fun-filled activity. If the weather is poor, put on your sneakers and take a walk around your local mall.

Friday: A Day for Hobbies

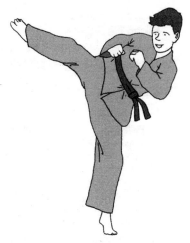

Help your children choose a hobby that can keep them physically fit.

For Friday, do something extracurricular with an instructor. There are many hobbies that involve physical activity. For example, you may take up martial arts, dance, or skating together as a family.

For Saturday Make Up Your Own Activity!

Make Saturday your free day. Pick something to do from the 52 Weeks of Fitness list (Figure 7.1). Here you will find enough activities to last you every Saturday for an entire year. You can also make up your own "fit activity" to do as a family on Saturday. The sky is the limit when it comes to exercise, so remember to keep moving!

Figure 7.1 *The Fifty-Two Weeks of Fitness*

Walking	House cleaning	Jumping rope
Throwing	Hiking	Dancing
Hopping	Frisbee	Crab kicks
Galloping	Soccer	Walk up stairs
Biking	Baseball	Body lunges
Curl-ups	Aerobics	Flexibility
Sprinting	Amusement park	Tumbling
Arm circles	walk	Swimming
Long jumps	Mall walk	Roller skating
Hula Hoops	Running	Gardening
Crab walks	Catching	Hockey
Running in Place	Skipping	Boating
Trunk turns	Jogging	Golf
Stretches	Pushups	Basketball
Yoga	Balancing on one	Football
Leg raises	foot	Playground play
Ice skating	Jumping jacks	Water park walk
Tennis	Toe touches	Skiing

The weekly exercise schedule outlined above is merely a suggestion to assist with your fitness planning. You need to take into account your child's likes and dislikes. I also recommend that your child's exercise plan include all members of the family. Remember, before you begin, everyone should be cleared for exercise by your family doctor.

CHAPTER EIGHT

Get in the Game:
Kids and Sports

Over the years I have heard many stories from parents and children, and seen for myself the achievements, failures, and frustrations of athletic competition. In this chapter I'll share some of these experiences to help you learn how to make your child's involvement in sports an enjoyable, lifelong hobby. I'll also discuss the parent's role in team sports, and what you can do to help your children engage in positive competitive activities. I'll also touch on the dos and don'ts of being a spectator or coach when your child is engaged in sports.

Being part of a team helps kids be active, cheerful and healthy, and can have a positive impact on them socially, emotionally, mentally and of course physically. The key to motivating your children to participate in sports is to provide a safe, comfortable and age-appropriate sports environment in which they can thrive.

Sports are physical activities that are governed by a set of rules, where individuals or groups develop skills to achieve a goal or objective through play. That's the text book definition. If only it were that easy! As many parents already know, sports become more and more complex as your children get older and more skilled, and while they can be an amazing outlet, they can also bring out the worst in human nature. Let's take a closer look at both the good and the bad of organized sports.

Sports are a great way for your children to have a good time while they engage in physical activity. Of course, sports don't always have to be about competition; they can be about spending quality time with family or friends without a thought given to who wins and who loses. Having a simple catch with your son or daughter can create a magical moment, the memory of which can last forever. Going to the yard or park and working on sport skills can help your children gain the confidence they may need to play with other children.

Team Sports

Competitive team sports can be a positive experience, but if supervised poorly they can be also have detrimental effects, not only for participants but also for spectators. Parents should be able to recognize any negative impact that competition may be having on their children. For example, if a child is playing on a basketball team that over-emphasizes winning, frustration and negative feelings among team members are often the result. Although striving to achieve goals is very important, working together to achieve that goal should occur in a fun environment that develops skills and engages all participants in a positive way. Let's examine the pros and cons of team sports.

The Pros

- **Sports improve social skills.** Having teammates can help our child make new friends. In some cases, your child will feel comfortable communicating with other children from his team because he is spending more time with them, and they now have something in common. It sets up a comfortable environment when he sees his teammates in other places such as school, recreation, or other extracurricular activities.

- **Sports reduce stress.** Playing sports in a relaxing setting can help children to relax and be happy. If they have a dominant, loud, forceful coach, of course the opposite result may occur. Mutual respect needs to be developed among everyone on the team to accomplish this objective.

- **Sports keep your children busy.** In many cases, when children are home, they are watching television, playing video games, or on the computer. Participation in team sports helps promote a healthy, active lifestyle now and in the future.

- **Sports help keep your children physically fit.** Many coaches work physical fitness routines into the sporting activity. During practices, coaches will work on the skills pertaining to the sport, but will also develop general fitness concepts.

- **Sports help improve cognitive skills.** Physical activity and exercise have been proven to help increase brain activity.

- **Sports teach children to work in group settings.** Many children are not comfortable working in groups, and prefer doing things individually. Sports can help these children develop social skills.

The Cons

- **Sports increase the chance of injury.** More children have the opportunity to hurt themselves in the heat of a battle. In some cases, children get hurt due to poor sportsmanship.

- **Sports involve the risk failure.** As mentioned earlier, make sure your children maintain a high degree of success whenever possible. But success should not just be measured by wins.

- **Sports can make children nervous about performance.** Many children worry about performing at high levels. When they fail, self-esteem and confidence can suffer.
- **Children often compare their skills to other children's skills.** Some children's self-esteem suffers because they feel they cannot compete with other children. The best way to combat this is to teach your children to always try to improve on their personal best.

The Parents' Role in Sports

Parents involved in sports play an influential role in their children's growth and development. Parents should never be looked upon as the enemy or the opposition, nor should a child feel nervous when participating in a sporting event in front of his parents. Rather, children should look to their parents as their strength and inspiration. By nature, a child wants to please his parents, so adding pressure will make this even more difficult to achieve, and may cause him to become discouraged and lose interest. As a parent of a child in sports, you take on several positive and important roles:

- **The Coach.** The parent is always a child's #1 coach. Your children might have coaches in school who change from year to year, but you are the consistent presence that they look up to.
- **The Educator.** From the day a child is born, parents become an influential mentor to them in all aspects of life, including physical activity. Your kids will learn an assortment of skills that will assist with their growth and development and boost their self-esteem.
- **The Nurturer.** Sometimes you win, sometimes you lose! There are a lot of emotions that come to the fore during competitive sports. Children need to accept every result thrown their way. You need to be compassionate and try to help your child deal positively with both victory and defeat.

- **The Mediator.** There may be conflicts with another child, parent or coach. Sometimes, you might need to be the intermediary to keep the peace.
- **The Fan.** Watching your children play a team sport can be very exciting. Remember, you're not there just to cheer your kids on to victory, but to encourage their efforts regardless of the outcome.
- **The Supporter.** Parents = Support, while Support = Parents. Always be there for your children.

Sportsmanship

Recently I was watching a basketball game between two young teams. All of a sudden, I heard one of the coaches yell out, "Damn it John, if you don't move your ass, I am taking you out of the game." There was a big hush over the crowd, and all the children stopped playing. The awkward silence seemed to last an eternity as the refs called a time out to talk with the coach. I could not hear what they were saying, but I assume it was, "Coach, please refrain from using that type of language with your players."

That coach may not have been aware of it, but he had just made a lasting, negative impression on the participants by showing both poor sportsmanship and generally poor behavior. Good sportsmanship is about fairness, determination, self-control, courtesy, integrity and a good overall attitude. Adults need to be the role models and educators when it comes to sportsmanship, or a sporting event may get ugly. Many children innately want to win at everything, while others are taught to just have fun and give their best effort. Regardless, parents need to enforce sportsmanlike rules that apply to all children, which will help create a comfortable atmosphere.

Parental Do's and Don'ts

- **Do** teach your children to be good sports.
- **Don't** be a bad sport yourself.
- **Do** teach your children not to argue with officials.
- **Don't** be a parent who argues with officials.
- **Do** teach your children to be gracious when they win or lose.
- **Don't** teach your children to show off if they win, or complain when they lose.
- **Do** teach your children to achieve personal best.
- **Don't** tell your children they did not play well, but build on the positives.
- **Do** teach your children to be constructive when they communicate.
- **Don't** teach your children to be rude and critical.

A Word about Age-Appropriate Activities

Sometimes parents put their children into an activity for which they aren't ready physically, socially or cognitively. There's no magical time at which a child is ready to participate in a particular sport. In many cases, it depends on the personality of the child, along with his or her maturity, physical skills, and confidence levels. It's up to both the parents and the child to decide when the time is right to participate in specific sports.

In general, very young children (ages 2 to 6) should engage in movement exploration activities and fewer competitive sports. Activities for this age bracket might include dance, tumbling, running, jumping, playground activities, bike riding, and walking. There's nothing wrong with working on various skills that will help develop fundamental sport skills such as throwing, catching or kicking. Once they have passed the age of 6, you can start to introduce your children to various sports, and the general rules and skills associated with them. This is also a great age to teach them about sportsmanship and about giving their best effort.

By age 8 or 9, children may start to play competitive sports, which can be modified according to their skill level. Be aware that this is a very impressionable age, as kids now start to compare their skills with other children's skills. By age 10, children will engage in more serious competitive sports, play on recreation or travel teams, and there is generally more emphasis on the outcome of the game and the contribution they have made to the team. By age 14 it will become even more intense, with longer workouts, traveling, and fitness training. It's important to keep in mind that, no matter what the age, participating in sports should be fun!

In the following pages I share some guidelines for healthy play in 10 different sports. I've chosen activities that focus on developing basic sports skills in a family environment. Feel free to modify some of the activities described to meet your interests and those of your children. These basic skills will serve as the foundation for future play with family and friends. Above all else, following these suggestions will increase your child's time being physically active, and that is the goal.

If you are not physically able to participate in these activities, it's important that you make the effort to watch your kids play, as this will motivate them to try harder. Again, both parents and children should be cleared by the family doctor before beginning these activities.

Len's Top Ten Sports Activities for Kids

1. **Basketball**
   a. Dribble Drill. Have your child dribble a ball to a designated area, then dribble the ball back. Have him maintain proper form: keep the ball about waist high while

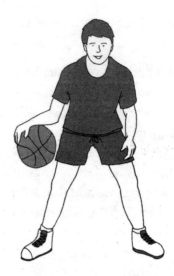

dribbling, use the fingertips for control, keep the head up and avoid slapping the ball with the palm of the hand.

b. **Chest Pass Drill.** Have your child pass the basketball to you or bounce it off a wall for one minute without rest. See how many passes can be made within that minute and then try to beat the score.

c. **20 Second Lay-Up Game.** A lay-up is a toss while standing very close to the basket. Give your child 20 seconds to make as many lay-ups as possible.

2. **Tennis**
   a. Practice serving the ball to each other on a tennis court or hardtop.
   b. Practice hitting the ball against a wall, both forward and backward swings.
   c. **Ball bounce.** Hit the ball approximately a foot in the air again and again. Do this as long as you can. Not much movement of the feet is needed if you do it correctly.

3. **Track**
   a. Practice sprinting 100 yards.

   b. Practice jumping over small hurdles while running.

   c. Throw a tennis ball as far as you can. Measure the distance, then throw it again, trying to beat your personal best.

4. Baseball and Softball

   a. Start with your child as the pitcher, and you as the catcher. After a while, switch spots.

   b. Practice running the bases.

   c. Practice hitting with yourself as the pitcher, and your child as the hitter. After a while, switch spots.

5. Football

   a. Try to throw the ball through a hanging tire or hula hoop.

   b. Practice throwing and catching.

   c. Practice running with the ball for an imaginary touchdown.

6. Soccer

   a. Have your child dribble the soccer ball to a designated area, then dribble back to the starting line.

   b. To increase accuracy, practice kicking the ball to a target.

   c. Take turns with a friend shooting a ball at a goal. First you child can be the shooter, then the goalie.

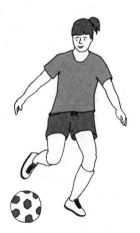

7. Boxing

   a. Like a boxer, jump rope in place. If you don't have a rope, go through the same motions with an imaginary rope.

   b. While jogging in place, practice jabbing back and forth as if you were a boxer.

c. Shadow box. You and your child face each other with one of you in the lead position: when you begin, the leader shadow boxes, while the other one mimics all the moves. After a few minutes, switch positions.

8. **Skiing**
   a. **Ski jump.** On "go," have your child jump back and forth between two spots for one minute.
   b. **360-degree jumps.** Have your child practice jumping in a complete 360-degree circle. From a starting position, he should jump and try to turn all the way around, landing in the starting position.
   c. **Practice balance by standing on one foot.** Hold that position for 20 seconds, then switch to the other foot.

9. **Volleyball**
   a. **Jump-ups.** Mark a spot on the wall with some tape and practice jumping up to touch it. Try doing it 20 times.
   b. Practice serving the volleyball over the net or to a wall.
   c. Practice hitting the volleyball over the net and aiming for targets on the ground on the other side, such as hula hoops.

10. **Hockey**
    a. Practice puck control to a specific area and return to the starting line.
    b. Practice shooting on goal.
    c. Practice passing the puck back and forth.

CHAPTER NINE

The World Is My Workout Buddy: School and Family Exercise Programs

I've been extremely successful in motivating millions of children to exercise. The secret to my success is simple: I design programs that make exercise fun, accessible, and rewarding. In this chapter I'll introduce you to ten novel programs I have designed that can be used as motivational tools to get children to exercise.

If you are going to be proactive about your children's health, that means doing your best to stay involved, even when they are at school. Talk to the principal and your kid's PE teacher and let them know that you want to make sure your children have the best foundation possible for a healthy future. You'd be surprised at how many schools want to get involved in fitness programs like those I've detailed below. It's also helpful to talk with other parents and get them involved. So do your best to persuade teachers, school administrators and other parents to put these programs in place. Go to your PTA meetings and be sure to speak up and explain your interest in these programs, which are of benefit to not only your own children, but every student in the school. By the way, don't forget that each of these programs can be adapted for use at home.

Len's Top Ten Exercise Programs

1. **Project ACES**

   Project ACES is an acronym for All Children Exercise Simultaneously, a program that takes place at the same time throughout the world on the first Wednesday in May. Begun 20 years ago in my own school in the state of New Jersey, it is now enjoyed by millions of kids around the globe.

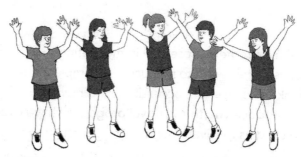

Project ACES
Millions of children exercise simultaneously each May

Back in 1989, as a PE teacher with classes in two schools, I was looking for a way to get my students motivated to exercise. At first, I thought it would be fun to get my kids in both schools exercising at the same time. Then I realized that, if I could get the kids in two schools exercising, I could get kids in every state to exercise at the same time and not only motivate children all over the United States to exercise, but also underline the importance of physical education in all schools. I began a letter writing campaign to schools throughout the United States, urging them to join in this exercise event.

When I first started, ACES stood for "American Children Exercise Simultaneously." There was no internet back then, so I needed to be creative in going about contacting schools. For example, if I wanted to recruit a school in Anchorage, Alaska, I would put information about ACES in an envelope and address the letter to the Anchorage Post Office. On the bottom corner of the envelope, I wrote in red ink, "Please deliver this envelope to any school in your district." I also put a self-addressed, stamped envelope in with the letter to make it easier for the schools to get back to me with an answer.

I had no idea if the post offices in any of the towns and cities I wrote to would actually forward it to a school, but they did. Almost everyone who received my letter thought joining in on ACES was a great idea and wanted to be part of it. I received confirmations day after day until every state had a participating school. The first year of ACES was a huge success. Children from 1,200 schools in all 50 states and from the island of St. Croix took part.

Within months of completing ACES 1989, I started receiving mail asking about the 1990 ACES event, which at the time did not even exist! Letters continued to pour in from schools throughout the country (almost 500 a day) and from outside the United States. It became obvious that the name of the program could not remain "*American* Children Exercise Simultaneously," and in 1990 it became "*All* Children Exercise Simultaneously." The first year of Project ACES, 240,000 children participated worldwide. Twenty years later, the state of Michigan alone had close to 500,000 participants and the project has received the praise of many people, including Presidents Bush and Clinton.

How It Works

Each year on the first Wednesday in May all the children in the program exercise, dance, walk, jog, participate in health clinics, bike ride, do aerobics, or a mixture of all of these activities. Each school organizes its own participation assembly. Schools and organizations can be as innovative as they would like in running the program for their kids. Many schools choose to invite local sport celebrities to the event, or play music to accompany the activities. Organizers of your local events can choose to get the entire school body involved, or just selected classes. The majority of schools will get the entire school population outside onto a playing field, put on music, and let everyone have some fun moving and exercising together.

If the weather is bad, some schools will have their kids do aerobics and calisthenics in the gym. Another option is to play music over the P.A. system and have the kids exercise in their classrooms. Some invite the local media to cover the event; the kids love to see themselves in the newspapers or on TV. In some instances, schools have had their town mayors and even state governors attend and read proclamations on fitness in honor of the event. Here are some examples of how easy it can be to organize an ACES Day event at your school.

Example 1: Fun and Simple Movement Activities

Total Time: 40 minutes

10:00 A.M.–10:05 A.M.: Light warm-up activities which include stretching exercises.

10:05 A.M.–10:10 A.M.: Light calisthenics that may include jumping jacks and running.

10:10 A.M.–10:15 A.M.: Heavy calisthenics that may include pushups and curl-ups.

10:15 A.M.–10:30 A.M.: Fun dances like the Chicken Dance, Macarena or the YMCA.

10:30 A.M.–10:40 A.M.: Slow walk as a cool down exercise.

Example 2: A Health and Fitness Fair
Total Time: 1 hour

10:00–11:00 A.M.: Create a health and fitness fair as a fun way to enjoy Project ACES Day. Set up exercise and health fitness stations around your school that the children will rotate around for 10 or 15 minutes, moving to the next station as the time expires.

Examples of stations:

a. Nutrition station. Have a local nutrition expert come in to discuss a healthy diet with the children. A presentation about healthy snacks makes a wonderful seminar. Samples make it even better!

b. Aerobics station. Have the local health club send one of their aerobics instructors to lead the kids in a workout routine.

c. Calisthenics station. Have the physical education teacher lead the kids in various calisthenics and dance routines.

d. Heart rate station. Have a representative from the American Heart Association teach the kids about monitoring their heart rate during activity.

e. Sleep station. No, not to rest, but an expert to discuss the importance of sleep in our daily lives.

f. Water station. A nutritionist leads a discussion about the importance of hydrating the body each day.

Example 3: Walking Activities

Total Time: 40 minutes

10:00 A.M.–10:40 A.M.: Set up a walking track around the school. The adult in charge should be able to account for all the children throughout the activity.

Example 4: Small Classroom Activities

Total Time: 15 minutes

10:00 A.M.–10:15 A.M.: Have each classroom in the school stop what they are doing and participate in some type of physical activity. They can follow any of the ideas above, or they can be creative and come up with their own.

The ways in which to organize this program are virtually unlimited. You have the flexibility to do whatever works best for you for as long as you wish; the duration of each activity depends on the school environment. The motivation for the participants comes from knowing that there are children and adults all over the world exercising along with them. Many schools throughout the country now have daily, weekly, or monthly Project ACES programs with different health, fitness, nutrition and lifestyle-related themes.

Project ACES Clubs

Since Project ACES started, the suggestion I've received most frequently is that it be held every day or at least once a week. This was how the idea of the Project Aces Club was born. Many schools have now organized ACES for every day, once a week or once a month, all leading up to the main event in May. We have designed the Project ACES Club so that kids can become members in four different categories: Platinum, Gold, Silver, or Bronze, through the ACES web site at www.projectaces.com. Here's how it works:

Platinum Member

Platinum members exercise every day in school or through their clubs or other organizations. Children volunteer to come in before school begins to exercise for 15 minutes with the teacher who is organizing the event. Or, a homeroom teacher may decide to do it each day with all the children in his or her classroom. If children have physical education class each day, their participation in those classes can count towards maintaining their Platinum member level.

Gold Member

Gold members exercise once a week in school. This may take place as part of a club before school, in the classroom or by participating in a weekly physical education class. It can also apply to an after school club that works with children in an ACES program once a week.

Silver Member

Silver members exercise once a month in school. The options for exercising are the same as for the Platinum and Gold members.

Bronze Member

This membership is popular with physical education teachers. To be a Bronze member, the child participates in a specific exercise for 15 minutes at the beginning of every physical education class.

2. **PACES Day**
   Each year after a successful ACES event, I received many letters and emails from parents asking me to create a program similar to ACES, but which includes adults. Finally, I did. PACES stands for Parents And Children Exercise

Simultaneously, and it takes place every weekend throughout the year, culminating on the first Saturday in May.

Children can enjoy Project ACES at school and also participate in PACES at home. PACES Day not only promotes exercise time, but family time. On PACES Day, parents exercise with their children for 15 to 45 minutes.

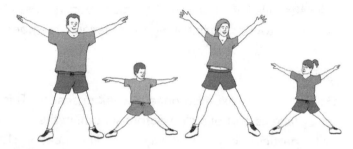

PACES encourages families to exercise together each weekend.

When you sign up for PACES Day online (www.pacesday .com), your family name is listed on the website along with all of the other PACES families from around the world, which is a great motivational tool to get your kids interested in participating. Here are 12 suggestions for enjoying PACES Day at home with your kids.

a. Take a Family Walk. Find a safe area in your neighborhood to take a family stroll. If the weather isn't cooperating, walk around the local mall for 30 to 40 minutes without stopping and just browse the shop windows. Remember, it's important to keep moving to get the most benefit.

b. Commercial-CIZE. This is a fun way to enjoy television together. Every time a commercial comes on, commit to performing a specific exercise. For example, during a show's first commercial break, the entire family should do 10 jumping jacks. For the next break, you may switch to performing 5 pushups. Try to get your kids to do this even when you are not watching with them. More on Commercial-CIZING later in the chapter.

c. **Exercise Videos.** Purchase an exercise video that is safe and fun for the entire family. Watch it as a family, and perform it as a family.

d. **Household Chores.** Working around the house is a form of exercise. As long as you create a safe environment, children can vacuum, rake leaves, take out the garbage, clean the garage, or paint a room.

e. **Family Hikes.** Find a safe, protected, and well marked hiking trail where you can take a family hike together. Put on the backpacks, hiking shoes, and pack a lunch for an exercise adventure.

f. **Bike Ride.** Find a safe area to take a family bike ride together.

g. **Theme Parks.** Take the children to a theme park. You have fun, but at the same time everyone does a lot of walking to all the attractions.

h. **Join a Local Gym.** Why not join a health club with your children? Some clubs offer discounts if the whole family signs up, and many offer exercise routines for children.

i. **Walk to School.** A great way to talk and exercise with your children is to walk them to school.

j. **Basic Calisthenics.** Teach your children the proper fundamentals for exercising properly. Show them how to do a pushup or jumping jack. Work on them together!

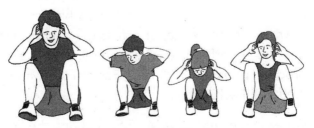

Basic calisthenics are fun to do as a family.

 k. **Eat Healthy Meals.** Your PACES event does not necessarily have to include only exercise. Why not plan on eating a very healthy meal each Saturday along with your exercise program?

 l. **Play Sports as a Family.** There are many sports you can do as a family, including basketball, baseball, football, hockey, soccer, gymnastics and tennis.

3. Exercise U.S.

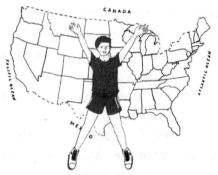

Children in the United States will exercise for 10 continuous hours.

Exercise U.S. (Exercise United States) takes place on the first Thursday in October. Like ACES, the idea behind the program is to motivate children to become healthy by making fitness fun. Children participate for 15 minutes in 10 continuous hours of fitness happening in countless locations from coast to coast. It works much like a relay race. Participating schools or organizations exercise their kids for 15 minutes at a set time during the day. Once completed, exercise begins at another school, which could be across town, across the state, or across the country, with its student body performing its fifteen minutes of exercise. The program begins at 8:00 A.M. Eastern time, and finishes at 3:00 P.M. Pacific time.

For example, at 8:00 A.M. (E.S.T.) during the first time slot of this program, a school in New Jersey begins to exercise.

This school will exercise for 15 minutes, ending at 8:15 A.M. At 8:15 A.M., a school in New York exercises until 8:30 A.M. At 8:30 A.M., another school, this time in Connecticut, begins exercising and concludes at 8:45 A.M. This pattern continues for 10 hours starting on the East coast and finishing on the West coast at 3:00 P.M. Schools can sign up to participate by visiting Exercise U.S. at www.uskidsworkout.com. One class or the whole school can participate, and more than one school or organization may sign up for a time slot. This program is a great way to highlight your school's physical education program or your organization's youth fitness program.

Examples of What You Can Do During an Exercise U.S. Event

The great thing about the Exercise U.S. program is that there are no set events in which kids must participate. Here are just a few suggestions for the Exercise U.S. event.

Walking

Try taking your children out for a brisk 15-minute walk around your school, YMCA or health club. Set up some cones to create a walking track and you will be all set to go!

Dance

Play your children's favorite dance music, anything from the Bunny Hop to the Macarena. The children will love dancing to the music.

Calisthenics

Exercises can range from running in place, to pushups, hopping, jumping jacks, and curl-ups, to name a few. Put it all to music and the kids will have a great time.

Jumping Rope

Jumping rope activities can be a lot of fun for 15 minutes. You can choose to have each child jump rope, or have them turning a longer rope for their peers.

Aerobics

Most local health clubs love to volunteer their time to visit a school and perform aerobics with the children. It's great publicity for the club and an opportunity for it to reach out to the community.

Yoga

Yoga is more than just stretching; it is about creating balance in the body through developing both strength and flexibility. Have the kids participate in a yoga class headed by a qualified instructor for 15 minutes during this event.

4. J Day

The concept behind J Day is simple: jumping jacks all day long for the whole school.

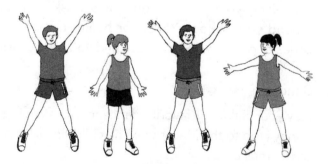

J Day will have children perform jumping jacks for an entire school day.

Jumping Jacks Day is very easy to organize and has a very high degree of success with kids. For our example, let's assume your elementary school has twenty classes and a seven-hour school day (8:00 A.M. to 3:00 P.M.). Figure 9.1 breaks down the day so each class can participate for 21 minutes in the event.

Figure 9.1 *J Day Organizing Formula*

A 7 hour school day = 420 minutes
There are 20 classes in our example

420 divided by 20 = 21

Each class will be responsible for 21 minutes of the program.

How Does J Day Work?

In our example, each class contributes 21 minutes to the day's event. Create a master schedule for the school to observe during the day. Figure 9.2 gives an example of how you might break down the classes for the day. Of course, many different ways to organize the day are possible.

Figure 9.2 *J Day Master Schedule*

Period 1	Period 2	Period 3	Period 4	Period 5
8:00–8:21	8:21–8:42	8:42–9:03	9:03–9:24	9:24–9:45
Class 1	Class 2	Class 3	Class 4	Class 5
Period 6	Period 7	Period 8	Period 9	Period 10
9:45–10:06	10:06–10:27	10:27–10:48	10:48–11:09	11:09–11:30
Class 6	Class 7	Class 8	Class 9	Class 10
Period 11	Period 12	Period 13	Period 14	Period 15
11:30–11:51	11:51–12:12	12:12–12:33	12:33–12:54	12:54–1:15
Class 11	Class 12	Class 13	Class 14	Class 15
Period 16	Period 17	Period 18	Period 19	Period 20
1:15–1:36	1:36–1:57	1:57–2:18	2:18–2:39	2:39–3:00
Class 16	Class 17	Class 18	Class 19	Class 20

Once your main schedule for the day is complete, get each class prepared for the program. First, sign each up for one of the periods in Figure 9.2. Once the classes are signed up, each teacher organizes the activity for the class' 21-minute period. If each class has 21 students, it may be difficult to have each class member perform jumping jacks for a full 21 minutes, so below are four alternatives for each class member's participation.

Alternative # 1

Have a baton handy. The children form a single line in the classroom. The first child in line performs jumping jacks for one minute. When done, he passes the baton to the next child, who does the same, until every child in class completes the task. Upon completion, the baton is passed to the next class to begin their portion of J Day.

Alternative # 2

Children can partner up and do the jumping jacks with their comrade for two minutes instead of solo for one minute. After that two-minute period, the baton is passed to the next pair. At completion, the baton is passed to the next class to begin its portion of J Day.

Alternative # 3

The kids can team up in groups of three and do the jumping jacks for a three-minute cycle before passing the baton to the next band of three. At completion, the baton is passed to the next class to begin its portion of J Day.

Alternative # 4

Team up the kids in groups of three again, but have them perform jumping jacks for one minute and then pass the baton over to the next group of three, who will do their allotment for one minute. When each group has completed its first minute of exercise, start the cycle again with the same groups of three for the next one-minute period, to be followed by the third and final one-minute period. At completion, the baton is passed to the next class.

These are just four options to consider. Obviously, there are many combinations you can explore for each grade level. You need to take into account the ages of your group members and the fatigue factor before you decide on an exercise format.

Organizing a J Day at Home with Your Family

You can easily modify the examples above to organize a J Day with your family at home. The plan need not be as involved as those described above. For our home example, we'll use a family of four, who are all healthy and medically cleared by their physicians to participate in this event. The time period for the entire event will be 28 minutes, as described Figure 9.3, say from 8:00 A.M. to 8:28 A.M.

Figure 9.3 *Family of 4—J Day Plan from 8:00 A.M. to 8:28 A.M.*

8:00 A.M.–8:01 A.M. — Dad does jumping jacks

8:01 A.M. –8:02 A.M. — Mom does jumping jacks

8:02 A.M. –8:03 A.M. — Child 1 does jumping jacks

8:03 A.M. –8:04 A.M. — Child 2 does jumping jacks

Repeat this process 7 more times

(You can use the alternative plans given earlier and modify them to meet your family's needs.)

5. Commercial-CIZING

TV has been called the "instant babysitter," and as both parents work longer days and need to keep the children occupied, they rely on TV more and more, a pattern that contributes to the overall poor fitness of our kids. How do you get kids to exercise without taking away their television privileges? Realistically, some parents should probably cut the amount of TV their children watch by half. The problem is, how do you monitor TV intake when you are working late and your child is responsible for himself when he comes home?

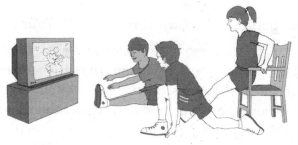

Why not have your children exercise during commercials?

Fortunately, about 8 to 10 minutes of each hour of television is devoted to commercials. What if your child commits to exercising every time a commercial comes on? I call this Commercial-CIZING. Here's how it works.

The formula in Figure 9.4 allows for a high degree of success with little chance of injuries. Use your discretion when choosing your exercises; they can be whatever your family agrees on. For repetitive exercises, an example would be 5 pushups per commercial. Two repetitions would be 5 pushups, rest, and then another 5 pushups per commercial. Assume your child is in 5th grade and watches four hours of television a night. He would be responsible for performing three repetitions of one or more exercises during

Figure 9.4 *Caption?*

Pre-K through Grade 1	One repetition of an exercise per commercial
Grades 2–3	Two repetitions of an exercise per commercial
Grades 4–5	Three repetitions of an exercise per commercial
Grades 6–8	Four repetitions of an exercise per commercial
Grades 9–12	Five repetitions of an exercise per commercial

each commercial break. He might do 25 pushups, 40 jumping jacks, and 50 arm circles. After finishing, he can relax and enjoy the show. When the next commercial break comes on, he begins again. He might do 25 curl-ups, 25 hops in place, and 25 no-rope jumping ropes.

You can also be creative about the activity your child performs. Instead of repetitions of exercises, your child can jog in place during the break, or have a healthy snack that includes fruits or vegetables. Let's do the math. If a child watches 2 hours of TV a day, that two hours includes about 30 minutes of commercial time. Those minutes can be used for exercise time. Please keep in mind that Commercial-CIZING is not meant to replace a regular exercise session, but rather enjoyed in conjunction with a child's established exercise routine.

6. **The Video Olympics**
   Can you imagine your school, organization, or family having a friendly fitness competition with another school, organization or family from your local area or from thousands of miles way? We'll, it is possible, and such a competition can foster an atmosphere in which kids can learn to enjoy fitness and exercise.

   In the late 1980's, I organized the first annual Video Olympics between Banyan Creek Elementary School in

Florida and New Jersey's Valley View Elementary School. The schools held a friendly competition in various exercises using simple videos that were exchanged through regular mail. The program proved to be a huge success, motivating hundreds of children to exercise. All you need is a video camera, email, and some motivated children.

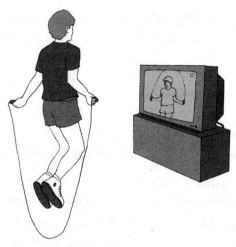

Fitness and technology working together!

The Video Olympics can be a competitive or non-competitive event, but the emphasis should always be on achieving one's personal best. If you choose the "getting a winner" route, try not to put too much importance on the competition (Figure 9.5) That is, no child should feel discouraged by his or her performance, and if scores are compared, the kids should compare their scores only with their own previous results in the competition, not with those of the other participants. One great benefit of the Video Olympics is the continuity factor: because the kids are filmed at least twice during the competition, they can compare their new scores to their past scores and follow their improvement in performance over time.

Figure 9.5 *For a Healthy Competitive Spirit*

- Try not to put too much emphasis on winning and losing. Keep the emphasis on doing one's personal best.
- Avoid elimination trials.
- Stress that sportsmanship is important.
- Focus on the skill at hand.
- Concentrate on learning the skill.
- Praise all kids equally.
- Remind kids that success is effort, and effort is success.
- If possible, make any competitive fitness activity voluntary.
- Create a fun, low pressure environment.

Here are a few suggestions to create both non-competitive and competitive but fun environments for the Video Olympics at home or in school. Choose the level you feel is appropriate for your child.

Level 1: Non-Competitive Level at Home

This is my favorite level of the Video Olympics, and the easiest to organize. It has a high degree of success and works with kids of all skill levels.

a. Pick one exercise, such as jumping jacks.
b. Set an objective. For example, the goal could be the most jumping jacks a child can perform in one minute.
c. Practice the proper fundamentals of the exercise to make sure your child is doing it correctly.
d. Train your child to be able to complete one minute of jumping jacks on a regular basis.
e. Pick a videotaping date with your child.
f. One that date, videotape your child performing jumping jacks for one minute.

g. Record his score.

h. Continue training for the event.

i. One month later, videotape your child again performing jumping jacks for one minute.

j. Compare the score from the previous video to see if your child has improved on his score. If yes, success. If no, just repeat the process, or try a new exercise. In most cases, a child will improve his score.

Level 2: Competitive Level at Home

At this level, a child competes with another child in a predetermined exercise. The children must agree on a training exercise and the exercise guidelines. This should be a voluntary activity, meaning a child should not be forced into this level if he doesn't want to compete.

a. Pick one exercise that both children agree on, such as pushups.

b. Set an objective for this exercise, such as the most pushups that can be performed until fatigue sets in.

c. Practice the proper fundamentals of the exercise to make sure the child is doing it correctly. At this level, a pushup that is completed incorrectly will not be counted in the total point score.

d. Train the child to be able to perform pushups on a regular basis.

e. Both children and their families should agree on a videotaping date.

f. On that date, videotape your child performing pushups until fatigue sets in.

g. Record his score.

h. Upload the video to your computer and send it to your child's competitor.

i. At the same time, your child's competitor emails his video to you. You can now compare your scores. Again, the emphasis should be on effort and sportsmanship.

Level 3: Non-Competitive Level at School

This is another very productive level of the Video Olympics. It has a high degree of success and also works with kids of all skill levels. It involves more children, and I have found that limiting the number of children that participate works best. When I organize this level, I do not to include the entire school population, in order to reduce the amount of time and videotaping involved. Instead, I form a Video Olympics afterschool club with about 15 children at most.

a. Pick an exercise, curl-ups for instance.
b. Set the objective, for example the most curl-ups the children can perform in one minute.
c. Practice the fundamentals of the exercise to make sure the children do it correctly.
d. Train the children to perform one minute of curl-ups on a regular basis.
e. Pick a videotaping date for all the children.
f. One that date, videotape all the children performing curl-ups for one minute.
g. Record their scores.
h. Continue training for this event.
i. One month later, videotape all the children again performing curl-ups for one minute.
j. Compare the scores from the previous video to see how many children improved on their score.

Level 4: Competitive Level at School

This level is more complicated than the previous levels, but exciting at the conclusion. In the finale, the Video Olympics pits the champions from one school or club against the champions from another. As always, the main emphasis is placed on the kids achieving their personal best scores.

Find another school or club that is willing to compete with yours. It could be a school in your town, or one across the country. For me and my kids, it is always more exciting the further away the competitor is. An easy way to find a school is to do an internet search, say, for elementary schools. Once you find another school, just email the PE teacher or fitness instructor. Many schools post the teacher's emails on their web pages. In my experience, most gym teachers are happy to be asked to take part.

Example of a Level 4 Video Olympics

Let's use a 9th grade high school class to demonstrate how this level of the Video Olympics is organized. First, select "challenge categories" in which your kids and the kids of the competing school will participate. For our example, the challenge categories could be pull-ups, pushups, curl-ups or jumping rope all performed in one minute. The goal is to perform the most of the selected exercise within the time limit chosen. The categories should be divided by gender to allow for both boy and girl winners in each category. Your winners will then be videotaped and the tape will be mailed or emailed to the competing school, which will videotape its winners and send it to you. The exchange of tapes should be completed on a predetermined date for fairness.

Before beginning, tell the children exactly how it is to be run. Explain the "challenge categories" with descriptions of how the event will be measured. Post signup sheets in the gym for each event and tell the children they can sign up on a voluntary basis for one event or more than one. Remember to obtain permission slips from the parents to allow the kids to stay after school to participate in their event.

When the day arrives to participate, watch how the children perform and record the scores. For example, you might have all the girls performing pull-ups first. After they finish, applaud their efforts and thank them for participating. The winner is the girl who does the most pulls-ups using the correct form. Depending on how many children sign up, you may have to extend this to a second or third day to finish.

When completed, you now have all your representatives to film for the finale of the Video Olympics. Now, here is the twist. I like to do a "call back" session. I invite all of the kids back a month later to try to improve on their initial score. This gets the kids working on the "personal best" aspect of competition. The majority of children who train will improve their score. I applaud all the children who attend the call back! I may even do call backs a few times throughout the year as a motivational tool.

The first part of the Video Olympics is now complete. Now that you have all of your winners in place, work with the school principal to have a school fitness assembly. The purpose of the assembly is to film the champions for the ultimate video exchange with the other school. All of the children who received the highest scores now perform their skill again with the video camera running. Invite the entire school population, parents, and administrators to watch these incredible performances by the children who are representing your school.

The Benefits of a School Assembly

- You can invite the local media to cover the event.
- The assembly is a non-competitive event, since you cannot see the children from the other school participate.

- It teaches great skills to the other students viewing the assembly.
- It shows the importance of good fitness habits.
- It puts physical education in the spotlight.
- It shows parents the significance of your program.
- It can motivate other children to exercise on their own.

Once you have all of your representatives videotaped, mail it to the other school on the predetermined date. The fun begins when you get the other school's video. It's a great opportunity to have a second assembly and show the results from the other school. For example, we would show the video of our boy who did the most pull-ups. Then we would show the video of the pull-ups champion from the other school to see if he achieved a higher or lower score.

7. 3-Exercise Challenge

The 3-Exercise Challenge ("3EC") is a unique program developed to measure the growth of a child's muscular strength and endurance while enhancing the participants' self-esteem. 3EC can take place at your local school, YMCA, recreation department or even at home.

The three basic components recommended for a 3EC program are pushups, curl-ups and pull-ups. However, you can decide which exercises to include.

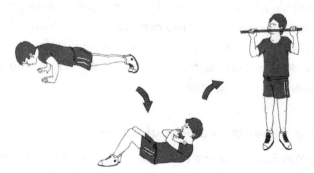

The 3-Exercise Challenge can include pushups, curl-ups, and pull-ups.

3EC may be considered a competitive activity, but it really depends on the approach you take when presenting it to your children, and in my view it is always important to put the emphasis on individual effort and achievement rather than getting the highest score.

How 3EC Works

3EC is an exercise marathon. Points are awarded for each successful exercise performed, so it is important to teach the kids the proper techniques of the three exercises before you start. Each participant has exactly three minutes to complete the program. Only one child at a time will execute the event, which is timed by the instructor. One minute is dedicated to each exercise. On the command of "go," a child begins the first exercise, which in our example is pushups. The child should do as many pushups as possible in the one-minute time allotment. The instructor awards one point for each successful pushup completed. A child may rest at any time.

When the first minute passes, the instructor must yell out a key word such as "switch" to start the next one-minute session, which are curl-ups. Again, a single point is awarded for each successful curl-up. A child may rest at any time.

As soon as one minutes passes, the instructor will once again yell out "switch" to start the third leg, which is chin-ups (if your facility or home does not have a chin-up bar, you may substitute a different exercise). The child is awarded one point for each successful chin-up completed. The child is finished with the event when he can no longer hang on the chin-up bar or if one minute passes. At this point, add up the final score (Figure 9.6).

Figure 9.6 *Example of a child's scorecard*

Minute 1: Pushups – 20

Minute 2; Curl-ups – 25

Minute 3: Pull-ups – 5

Total Points = 50

It is essential to create a safe environment for this event. As mentioned, a child may rest at any time without being penalized. It is also important to select a proper location in your school or home to perform the program. Safety mats are highly recommended for all three exercises.

If doing 3EC at home, first find out if your child is interested in participating. You don't want to force him to participate if there is no interest. As long as you can create a non-pressured environment, most kids will play. If 3EC takes place at school, you must decide if you want all the children to participate or just those who are interested. I recommend that participation in this event take place on a voluntary basis at school for two principal reasons. First, the individual performances can be lengthy, which creates prolonged limited activity for the remaining students in the class. Second, of course, is that no child should be forced to participate in an event in which he or she has no interest.

Types of Competition

Approach 1: Individual Competition

The first type of competition for the 3EC is the individual level, and the one that I recommend for this activity, since the children do not compete with their peers; rather, they challenge themselves to achieve personal best scores. In my experience, children are more motivated to enhance their personal best skills than when they are competing against kids who may be gifted physically. This type of competition works better if you do it at home.

Approach 2: Comprehensive Competition

You may decide to have the children compete against one another in a formal competition. If you choose this approach, I recommended that it be done on a voluntary basis so as to place the least amount of pressure on kids who may feel uncomfortable with the contest. You must also decide if you want to get a single winner from your school, or get divisional winners using categories. Categories can include age, gender, grade or class.

8. Map Moving

With Map Moving, all you need is a plan, a map, and a family determined to walk. When your family walks a predetermined distance each night, they accumulate miles on a map. The family sets a goal for themselves, and when they reach their goal, they create a family prize such as going to the movies, a family hike or out to dinner.

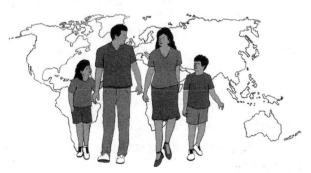

Walk around the world with your family. It is great physical activity and educational.

Imagine a family of five that lives in the United States. They create their "map goal" of walking the entire the country. There are two ways to go about this: one is by "collecting" all 50 states, the other by walking from the east coast to west coast, or vice versa. Of course, if you do not live in the United States, make up your own challenges for your own country.

Collecting All 50 States

For each night you take your walk and meet your objective, you collect a state. Your objective is whatever your family determines it to be. For example, your family might have a goal of walking two miles each night.

Hang a map of the United States on your refrigerator door, or just a list of all the states on a plain piece of paper (Figure 9.7).

For each day you reach your walking objective, cross off a state on your map or list. Once you reach your goal of all 50 states, your family should reward itself with something special.

Moving From East Coast to West Coast

Similar in concept to the above, but instead of collecting a state when the family meets its objective, they mark off a specific distance on the map. Suppose the map you have is 12 inches wide. Each time a family meets its objective, it moves from east to west 1/3 of an inch. The goal may be to start in New York, and end in California. Again, when they meet their final objective, a family reward should be enjoyed by all.

Figure 9.7 *Collect the 50 states*

1.	Alabama	26.	Montana
2.	Alaska	27.	Nebraska
3.	Arizona	28.	Nevada
4.	Arkansas	29.	New Hampshire
5.	California	30.	New Jersey
6.	Colorado	31.	New Mexico
7.	Connecticut	32.	New York
8.	Delaware	33.	North Carolina
9.	Florida	34.	North Dakota
10.	Georgia	35.	Ohio
11.	Hawaii	36.	Oklahoma
12.	Idaho	37.	Oregon
13.	Illinois	38.	Pennsylvania
14.	Indiana	39.	Rhode Island
15.	Iowa	40.	South Carolina
16.	Kansas	41.	South Dakota
17.	Kentucky	42.	Tennessee
18.	Louisiana	43.	Texas
19.	Maine	44.	Utah
20.	Maryland	45.	Vermont
21.	Massachusetts	46.	Virginia
22.	Michigan	47.	Washington
23.	Minnesota	48.	West Virginia
24.	Mississippi	49.	Wisconsin
25.	Missouri	50.	Wyoming

9. Fitness Pen Pals

It is always great idea to work on fitness and cognitive skills together. Many studies have shown that a solid exercise program enhances a child's intellectual well-being. It is also true that by enhancing cognitive skills, you can strengthen physical performance. This is one of the innumerable reasons why physical education in the schools is vital, and why the push for children's fitness is becoming so intense at health clubs.

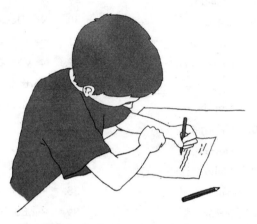

Pen pals can share fitness challenges through the mail.

Fitness Pen Pals is great for combining mental and physical fitness. A child from one location will write to another child in a different area by mail, which in my experience is more effective, and more easily supervised than email. Usually, it is arranged between a teacher or parent from one location with a teacher or parent from the other location (this also promotes a safe affiliation). In a school, the Fitness Pen Pal program is a great way for a classroom teacher to team up with the school PE teacher. It makes education fun as children learn to exercise *and* improve their writing skills.

Fitness Pen Pals is also an enjoyable program for parents to do with their children at home. You may want to participate with a neighbor, or a relative that lives a distance away. In fact, this program is probably easier to develop for a parent at home than a teacher at school.

Generally, when pen pals communicate, they share information about their school or environment. For instance, if a child in Maine is writing to a child in Florida, information can be shared about the different weather found in each state. Other topics could include:

- What is your favorite subject?
- What sports do you like?
- What are your favorite professional teams?
- Do you have any pets?
- Do you exercise a lot?

Now let's toss fitness skills into the mix. The pen pals ask the usual questions, but at the end of their letters, include a realistic fitness challenge. For example, a participant may write at the end of her letter, "I challenge you to perform 25 pushups every day for one week." The receiver must try to live up to this challenge as best he can! One child may not write another letter (challenge) to her Pen Pal until she receives one in return from her Pen Pal. It must alternate to work properly!

Organizing Fitness Pen Pals

Most teachers love when a parent volunteers to assist with a unique program in the classroom. It makes it easier for them, but also brings in fresh ideas. In this section, we will look at an 8th grade middle school class participating in the Fitness Pen Pals program. To begin, explore the possibilities of attracting another school to participate. This may be a challenge, especially if you would like to find a school that is far away. Here are four ways to find another 8th grade class from a different school to join in. These four methods can be used for any grade level.

Pen Pal Method 1: The Internet Route

You can do a search on the Internet to find another school. Use the terms "middle school," "junior high school," "8th grade" or "intermediate school" for your search. Most schools have their own websites with all of the contact information you'll need. Once you find a desirable school, contact it to find out if it would be interested in participating.

Pen Pal Method 2: The Post Office Path

Suppose your 8th grade class in New Jersey wanted to get a school in Anchorage, Alaska to participate in the program. How can you do this? Here's a technique that worked for me. On a business size envelope, put your return address in the upper left-hand corner. In the delivery address, write the following: Anchorage Post Office, Anchorage, Alaska 99501. In the lower left-hand corner write the following: Dear Post Office – Please Deliver This to an 8th Grade School.

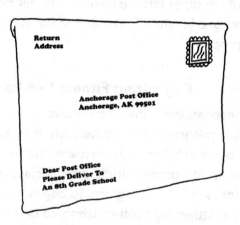

To get a zip code of a town or city, you can search on the internet. Your letter should include information about the Fitness Pen Pals and a request that the school join in. You should include your name, school address and phone for them to contact you with their answer.

Pen Pal Method 3: The University Student Teacher Circuit

Most major colleges or universities have physical education departments. Follow the same procedure as above. As the address, write the following: The University of Anchorage, PE Department, Anchorage, Alaska 99501

Include in your letter information about the Fitness Pen Pals program. Ask the recipient to pass the letter along to any student teachers working at the middle school level. The letter should ask the student teacher's school if it would like to join your school in the Fitness Pen Pals program. You should include your name, school address and phone number to receive an answer.

Pen Pal Method 4: The Friends and Family Route

Simply ask colleagues, family members or friends if they know of anyone outside of your area who might want to participate in the Fitness Pen Pals program. Once you get a lead, make contact with them about the event.

Regardless of the method you choose to use, once you have a school agree to participate, it is important that you exchange names. Write up class lists and mail them to the supervising adult at the other school. It is recommended that you use first names along with the last initial for safety reasons. For example, you would send a list of names to the corresponding school as follows: Gina P., Max R., Evan S., Loretta C., Rita S. and so on. Once you get your list from the other school, write down individual names on an index card with the corresponding address and pass them out to your participants to begin their letter writing campaign.

Monitoring

Since part of this program takes place outside of your school or club environment, you must do the best you can to monitor the program. This is for the safety of all involved. You will have to talk with your building administrators to go over a safety plan. Here are a few precautions to consider:

a. Get written parental permission for each child's participation.
b. Use the school mailing address at first. The mail should be addressed to the child, care of the teacher.
c. Try to read all outgoing and incoming letters.
d. The teacher should mail the letters once they are examined.
e. Supply examples to the children on what to write.
f. If the child wants to use her home address after a period of time, she must bring in a separate permission slip to do so.
g. Tell the child not to write any letters confidentially.

10. **The Exercise Video**

How many parents have purchased some type of exercise video to get fit at home? Probably many of you have. For many it works wonders; for others, it just collects dust on a shelf.

What about creating your own fitness video, starring you or your kids? Before you start laughing, it may actually work for you! Videotaping is simple. Your children would love exercising daily to a video that they actually made or starred in, and it is very easy to do.

First, create a script. Come up with some type of exercise routine that may involve dancing, aerobics, calisthenics, yoga or all the above. Once the script is completed, have your child practice the routine before film time. Of course, keep in mind that they are actually exercising while practicing!

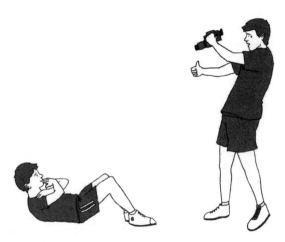

Home exercise videos can be a lot of fun!

When everyone is comfortable with his or her routine, it is film day. Videotape you or your children performing the routine. When the tape is completed, they can now follow it every day to get exercise, whether you play it on the television or the computer. This can be hours of fun and great exercise. Give it a try.

CHAPTER TEN

Make a Rainy Day an Active Day

Bad weather doesn't mean that physical activity must come to an end. In this chapter, I'll give you some ideas to keep the blood pumping on poor weather days.

When I was a kid living in a large apartment building minutes outside of New York City, my friends and I spent virtually all of our time in the city park just behind the building, where we played basketball, stickball, baseball, football, hockey and tennis. Even on rainy days you could find us in our ponchos in that park. But when the weather was so bad we had to stay inside, we would come up with creative ideas to keep ourselves busy. Whether it was tag in the hallways, jogging up and down the steps, mock basketball in the lobby or wall ball in the laundry room, we were still active. Sometimes it was more fun playing inside than it was playing outdoors. Here are 25 activities you and your kids can enjoy regardless of the weather.

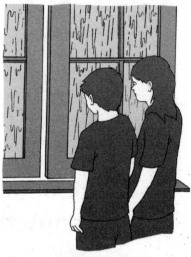

Kids don't have to be inactive on rainy days!

1. **Mall Walking**

   This is a great activity to keep your family active. Malls have large open spaces in which to walk, as well as steps to go up and down. Visit your local mall, lay out a walking circuit, and you are all set. Time yourself walking your course, then try to beat your time on the next circuit. Of course, the window shopping helps make the circuit interesting.

2. **Look For Indoor Play Gyms in Your Area**

   Recently, many enclosed facilities have begun to include basketball courts, baseball or soccer fields, rock climbing and even swimming. Look online or in your local yellow pages to find one in your area. These facilities have become very popular for children's birthday parties, and are also open all year to the public.

3. **Make an Exercise Video**

   As mentioned in the previous chapter, it's easy to make your own exercise video. Most digital cameras now have a feature which allows you to upload your video to your computer and exercise to your own routine. This can be a lot of fun for the whole family and your child's creativity and personality get a chance to shine.

4. **Go Bowling**

   Bowling is a fun family activity. It develops eye-hand coordination, aiming, and muscle strength, and keeps your kids away from the TV as well.

5. **Fun Dances**

   Find silly movement activities that are fun like "the chicken dance" that are easy to "shake it" to and great indoor enjoyment. You can listen to many of these songs free online at various web sites geared towards children.

6. **Indoor Exercise Scavenger Hunt**

   Create a list of things to hide around the house. With each object, place a tag on it with a specific exercise. For example, let's say a tennis ball is one of the objects to find. Attach a note to it that says, "Five pushups." Whoever finds the tennis ball keeps the object, but must also perform 5 pushups before they look for the next object. Do this with the rest of the objects hidden around the house. When complete, start over again, hiding the objects in different places in your house. It's a lot of fitness fun!

7. **Jumping Rope**

   If you have a high enough ceiling, jumping rope can be a lot of fun in most rooms of your house. Set a one minute time limit, and see how many jumps each family member can do in that time frame. If your family doesn't have any rope, practice the exact movement without the rope. You can also play the "snake game." One person holds the rope while standing in the middle of the room (furniture should be moved to the sides). The person holds only one end of the rope, while letting the other end lie on the floor.

The person begins to spin in a circle carefully while holding one end of the rope so the other end begins to move in a circle. The "twirler" must keep the rope spinning at ground level. At this point, all the other family members move close to the spinning rope and jump over it with each pass.

8. **Create a Family Exercise Routine**

   As a family, sit down at the kitchen table and have each member create 5 different exercises. Put them in any order you like. Pick some fun, upbeat music that you all love, choreograph it to the music, and start your routine. Each week, add new exercises to the existing routine to make it longer. After a few days of practice, this could be something your family can do every day, rain or shine, to stay healthy and fit together.

9. **Walk the Stairs**

   If you have stairs in your house, practice walking up and down your stairs as many times as you can in one minute. The little ones should use the handrails. You can also use the bottom step only to practice step aerobics. Step up with your right foot on the bottom step, and then the left foot must go up to the same step. From there, the right foot goes back down to the ground level, followed by the left foot. Continue this pattern for a set amount of time. Always make sure your children are properly supervised.

10. **Indoor Obstacle Course**

    If your family is creative, you can set up a fun obstacle course using the entire house. On "go," start by doing 5 jumping jacks in the kitchen. Run to the living room and jump through 4 hula hoops. From there, run to the bathroom, and jump up and down 10 times. Once done, run up the steps to the master bedroom and do 5 pushups, then go back to the kitchen and drink a glass of water. Your family will have a lot of fun with this. Just make sure safety is discussed before you start.

11. Hula Hoops

Hula hoops can be a lot of fun for the family. Not much room is needed, and you can practice twirling the hoop to music with it around your waist, neck, or arms. You can even jump rope with a hula hoop.

12. Mirror Exercises

Here's how it works. For example, a mother and father face each other about 5 feet apart. Whatever the mother does, the father must mirror: when the mother does 5 pushups, the father mimics this movement. Then the mother may perform 10 jumping jacks; the father must follow suit. After a few minutes, the pair should switch the leader so everyone gets a chance to use his or her imagination.

13. Balloon Activities

Balloons can be a lot of fun, and they are safe to use inside. Practice throwing and catching the balloons, or play balloon tennis. Put some tape on the floor to mark out a "net" and "foul lines," get some tennis rackets and have some fun.

14. Family Yoga

Put on some relaxing music and start to practice breathing exercises, meditation, and healthy physical postures. Working on safe stretches will also relax the family and keep everyone's mind off of the horrible weather taking place outside.

15. Balance Activities with Bean Bags

Beanbags are great for working on balance and posture; you can find them in many of your local dollar stores. Try walking around your house with a beanbag balanced on your head; try going up and down the steps without using your hands to hold it in place. Try other fun ways to balance the beanbags, like placing it atop the laces on your shoes, and walking around the house. You could even try to play beanbag tag, where one family member is "it" and must chase other family members around the house. All participants must balance the beanbags on their heads while playing: no holding the beanbags with your hands! When someone tagged, he must do 10 jumping jacks before returning to the game.

16. **Throwing and Catching with a Bean Bag**

Beanbags are a fun and safe way to work on your child's throwing and catching skills; you can even set up a mock bowling alley using old soda bottles and aim the bean bags at the bottles to see who can knock over the most in 10 rounds. You can be creative and play a clapping game with the beanbags: stand still and toss the beanbag in the air, then catch it. Then follow the same pattern, but while the beanbag is in the air, clap one time before catching it. If successful, follow this pattern but clap two times. Keep going to see how many claps everyone can do without missing the beanbag.

17. **Join a Local Indoor Pool Club**

Swimming is a great way to exercise. Many town recreation centers or YMCAs have indoor pools where you can swim any time of the year. Some facilities offer free or inexpensive swim lessons, which are great exercise in themselves. Participating on a swim team is great training if your child enjoys the water.

18. **Exercise with Video Games**

Some video games require children to dance, play music, or exercise along with the game. This type of technology is welcome on poor weather days.

19. Simple Calisthenics

Put on some music and try some simple exercises as a family such as pushups, curl-ups, jogging in place, jumping rope, jumping jacks, toe touches or mountain climbers.

20. Household Chores

Rainy days are great for organizing or cleaning up your house. Kids can vacuum or sweep the floor for some great exercise, as well as dust the rooms and clean the windows.

21. Exercise Shows on TV

There are now many exercise shows on television that you can follow to help stay fit. Check your local listings to find the times and enjoy exercising with the professionals. Please keep in mind that some of the exercises may not be appropriate for children, so use your best judgment.

22. Exercise Websites

The internet is a valuable tool to find health web sites that teach children quite a bit about health, including the proper mechanics of various exercises and good nutrition. Do a simple search such as "exercise for children" or "nutrition for children," and you'll get many worthwhile results.

23. Simple Tumbling on a Thick Blanket

Parental supervision will be needed to make sure your children are careful performing basic tumbling skills on a very soft, thick blanket. Such skills as rolling, forward roll and leapfrog can be safe fun on a rainy day. Be creative and careful.

24. Hopscotch in Your Garage

Set up a hopscotch game in your garage if you have the room, or create a hopscotch court using tape in your home. This can provide hours of fun.

25. Commercial-CIZE

Exercise during commercials. No doubt on rainy days your children will watch more TV, so have them exercise when the commercial breaks come on.

These are just a few suggestions for your family to follow. Many of the activities require very little equipment, so your costs will be low. It's important to put safety first and create an environment with proper supervision where there is no chance of injury. Use your best judgment in what you do and enjoy.

Okay, we've learned how to motivate kids to get moving and stay fit, and we've discussed great, fun ways to keep them involved in their own health. But there's more! Let's address some of the fundamentals of health such as nutrition, hydration and sleep, which will keep your kids energized and enjoying the benefits of good health now and into the future.

PART THREE

Your Child's Inner Fitness: Nutrition, Hydration and Sleep

CHAPTER ELEVEN

Fuel for Fitness: Proper Nutrition and Healthy Snacking

You may recall your own parents saying to you, "You are what you eat." This adage is actually quite true. If you eat unhealthy foods, you're probably not going to perform at your highest level, and will feel generally run down. Your brain and your body need food for fuel!

It's important to educate your kids about the benefits of healthy eating. However, most children feel healthy and energized naturally, and the logic that might convince an adult, that one should eat right and exercise to feel healthy, simply does not make sense to a child. Another strategy is needed with kids. Earlier, we discussed the "bank method" of teaching your children about exercise, and it can also be applied to eating habits. Simply put, eating healthy as a young child will pay off with many positive health dividends later in life, just as putting money in the bank makes you financially stronger at a later time.

Simple changes in your family's diet can make a big difference in your children's health. Many of these changes require little effort, and are quite easy to follow. First, let's explore the food groups and discover how important they are to your children's health (and yours). Then I'll suggest some kid-approved snacks, and entire meals as well, that are delicious, healthy and, best of all, fun.

The Healthy Food Groups

Carbohydrates, Proteins and Fats

The energy we obtain from food comes from carbohydrates, proteins, and fats in the form of calories. These energy sources are known as macronutrients and they are essential for the proper growth and development of your child. The United States Department of Agriculture recommends that 50 percent of total caloric intake come from carbohydrates, 20 percent from protein, and 30 percent from fat.

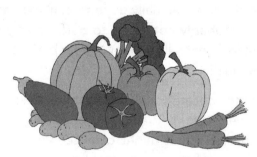

Teach your children to eat healthy foods while they are young.

Carbohydrates

There are the two types of carbohydrates: simple and complex. When carbohydrates are digested, they enter the bloodstream and are converted to "body fuel" called glucose. How fast the carbohydrates enter the bloodstream and become glucose depends on the type of carbohydrates that are ingested and whether there was fiber, protein or fat in that meal. Complex carbohydrates are digested slowly, keep you feeling fuller longer and provide a more steady flow of energy to the body. They should provide the majority of the energy your child needs each day. Examples of good sources of complex carbohydrates are whole grains such as oatmeal, oat bran, whole wheat breads, pastas, buckwheat (kasha), quinoa, barley, spelt, beans and lentils. These carbohydrates provide lasting energy, fiber, vitamins and minerals naturally.

Simple carbohydrates, on the other hand, tend to be highly processed, contain fewer nutrients and tend to be less filling and more fattening. Simple carbohydrates are broken down by the body much more quickly if consumed without any other macronutrients, and can give your child an energy spike, possibly followed by an energy crash.

A few examples of simple carbohydrates are table sugar, soda, cakes, cookies, and candy, all of which are processed foods. If a child eats nothing but fruit juice and donuts for breakfast, they are eating far too many simple carbohydrates, which perpetuate persistent sweet cravings. Remember, the closer foods are to their unprocessed, natural state of composition, the better they are for you!

Protein

Protein is used by the body to make enzymes, which assist in the building and repairing of cells. Protein regulates a vast number of bodily functions, including helping the nervous system to send and receive messages to and from the brain. Proteins also assist the immune system in fighting off disease and infection. Simply put, protein is important to building stronger muscles, bones, and organs. Protein also plays an important role in keeping your skin and tissues healthy.

Protein comes from two sources: plant and animal. Complete proteins come from animal sources such as meat, chicken, and fish, eggs and dairy, but may also be found in soybeans. Complete proteins carry all the essential amino acids the body needs. Incomplete proteins do not. They are, however, readily available in plant foods such as nuts, seeds, vegetables, grains and beans. Vegans who eat a variety of grains, legumes and vegetables can easily create meals with plenty of complete proteins to meet or exceed the body's protein requirements.

Animal protein can be associated with a higher fat content, and consuming too much can contribute to an increased risk of high blood pressure, heart diseases and high cholesterol. Vegetable protein sources are generally healthier because they contain good sources of dietary fiber and generally a much lower fat content, particularly the unhealthy saturated fats. For example, one ounce of almonds provides 6 grams of protein, nearly as much as one ounce of rib eye steak, and almonds are an excellent source of essential fatty acids!

Fats

Fats enhance the flavor, texture and extend the shelf life of many foods. Fat is an essential nutrient (a nutrient that must be obtained from food) that provides energy, insulation, organ protection, hormone balance, regulates body temperature and keeps your skin and hair healthy. The body will store all excess energy (calories) as fat, and we have an endless capacity for storage. Fat deposits surround and protect organs such as the liver, kidneys, and heart. Fats are necessary to transport and absorb vitamins A, D, E and K. It's essential to have some fats in your diet to maintain normal body functions.

There are four main types of fats: monounsaturated fat, polyunsaturated fat, saturated fat and trans fats. Mono and polyunsaturated fats are the "good" fats. Saturated and trans fats should be avoided or consumed in moderation.

Saturated Fats.   Saturated fats are those that are solid at room temperature. They are found mostly in animal products such as meat, turkey, chicken, dairy products (except skim and fat-free), butter, fried foods and lard. Processed foods such as cakes, biscuits, ice cream and coffee creamers are made using hydrogenated vegetable oils, which are saturated fats. Too much saturated fat in the diet can lead to heart disease and high blood pressure.

Trans Fats.   As of January 1, 2006, all food labels were required to state the amount of trans fat present in the food item. When this happened, many food processors, which used trans fats to extend the shelf life of their products, rapidly reformulated their products to remove the trans fats. This was for very good reason: trans fats are truly a health hazard! Trans fats increase triglycerides and LDL cholesterol (bad cholesterol) and reduce HDL (good cholesterol). The body cannot effectively break down trans fat molecules, which in turn raises cholesterol levels and reduces our own shelf life.

Unsaturated Fats.   There are two types of unsaturated fats: mono and polyunsaturated. These healthy fats remain liquid at room temperature. They are found mostly in plant products including nuts and seeds and are also found in fish and many oils. Using these types of fats in your diet, as opposed to saturated fats, can actually help lower your cholesterol and blood pressure levels. Examples of monounsaturated and polyunsaturated fats are olive and peanut oils, nuts and nut products like almond and peanut butter, and cold water fish such as salmon (which is also rich in heart-healthy Omega 3 fatty acids). However, as with all things in our diet, moderation is imperative.

Essential Fatty Acids.   Essential fatty acids (EFAs) are the kind of dietary fats that help promote good health. Omega 3 and Omega 6 are the two most important types of EFAs. You will find these essential fatty acids in foods such as olive and flaxseed oils, walnuts, soybeans, safflower and sunflower oils, salmon, tuna and sardines. You might ask what makes these oils "essential". They are critical for eye, brain and several other neurological functions. The EFAs also help to lower LDL (bad) cholesterol.

Vegetables, Fruits, and Dairy Products

We've briefly covered all the macronutrients and where to find each in our food supply. Vegetables, fruits, and dairy products are just as important to include in your child's diet. They are some of the most important food groups available to supply us with the nutrition we need every day. Vegetables are an excellent source of carbohydrates and provide many of the vitamins and minerals kids need for optimum health. They are low in calories, high in water content, and provide fiber, which helps us feel full and lowers cholesterol. Did you know that dark green leafy vegetables (such as kale, collard greens and spinach) provide fiber, vitamins and minerals like calcium and iron?

Fruit is nature's candy! Fruits are rich in minerals, vitamins, carbohydrates and fiber. They are also high in water content, which is an important contributor to keeping your children hydrated throughout the day. Fruits help stimulate the memory, they are low in calories, contain fiber, are inexpensive and taste great.

When choosing veggies and fruits for your family, try to include as many colors as you can find! Eat all the colors of the rainbow. Not only will your child's plate look more appetizing, but he will be eating a wide variety of essential nutrients.

Dairy products are good sources of protein, calcium, potassium, phosphorus, riboflavin, vitamin A and vitamin D. The dairy group can be one of the largest contributors to calcium intake, which is extremely important for bone health. Many dairy products can be high in saturated fats, since they come from animals, so choose low fat or fat free products to lower cholesterol intake and fat content when you can. Low fat yogurt tastes just as good as regular yogurt, and has the same nutrients, but without the saturated fat which can clog your arteries!

Be sure your child has food choices available each day from all macronutrients: carbohydrates, proteins and fats. Remember to include whole grains, plant sources of protein and healthy fats in your child's daily diet. Keep a wonderful and colorful variety of vegetables and fruits on hand and readily available to your child. Always choose whole, natural, unprocessed foods over refined foods whenever available. And remember to help your children make good choices by choosing healthy foods for yourself. Your body will thank you, and your children will thank you by being strong and healthy!

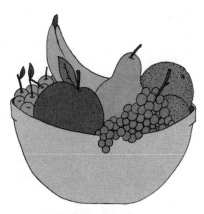

Make wise choices for your children's snacks.

Mind Those Snacks!

In many households, parents have some control over what their children have for meals. But most problems occur with eating between meals, when children frequently binge on unhealthy snacks. Once again, it is your responsibility to educate your children about better snack foods. Keep your house stocked with better options, and keep the junk and high fat snacks out of your home. Below are recipes for delicious, healthy snacks your children will love, and I've also given you some healthy meal suggestions. Remember, if you help your children to moderate their snack timing and volume, they will eat their meals. Give them better choices and you'll see better results.

Len's Top Ten Tips for Healthy Snacking

1. Give the children better choices.
2. Reduce snacks before meals.
3. Limit snacks with excessive added sugar.
4. Allow children to pick their own healthy snacks.
5. Eliminate non-nutritive beverages (sugary sodas, artificial fruit juices)
6. Control snack portions.
7. Avoid serving processed foods and those made with artificial sweeteners.
8. Provide your child with a morning and afternoon snack each day.
9. Include vegetables or fruits in every meal or snack. Try to eat at least 5 servings each day of fruits and vegetables combined.
10. Remember, children are not mini adults, so when you serve a meal, a child's portions should be appropriate to his size and age

Easy Recipes for Healthy Snacks

Your children will love these healthy snacks, and they are so much better for them than the snacks they are used to which are no doubt full of sugar, salt and fat.

Frozen Banana Slices

This is a simple, easy to prepare, healthy snack. Slice a banana and place each slice on a plate without stacking them. Cover the plate with aluminum foil and leave it in the freezer for 2 hours. After 2 hours, enjoy your snack. Your children can eat them as individual slices, or place some on a plate and mush them together to eat with a spoon. The snack is high in potassium and fiber.

Frozen Yogurt Sticks

Most children like yogurt, and it is an excellent source of calcium and protein. Many of the major companies now have liquid versions of yogurt so children can easily drink it. It's fun to freeze the yogurt and eat it like an ice pop. Simply pour a yogurt into a paper cup and place tin foil over the top. Stick an ice cream stick through the middle of the foil to hold the stick in place while it freezes. Take it out after a couple of hours and enjoy!

Pizza Muffins

Most kids will pick pizza as one of their favorite meals. How about pizza on a high fiber or whole grain muffin? All you need is some muffins, low-fat shredded mozzarella cheese, sliced tomatoes, and a toaster oven. Lay some of the muffins on foil and place a slice of tomato on top of each muffin. Sprinkle some of the cheese on top of the tomato and place in the toaster oven for a few minutes. Instant healthy pizza snack! An excellent source of calcium, complex carbohydrates, potassium, and vitamins A and C.

Fruit Kabob

Does your child have a favorite fruit or two? Why not make them fruit kabobs? Cut up their favorite fruits; push a wood skewer through the fruit, and have instant fun eating a healthy snack full of vitamins and minerals.

Rice Cake Sandwiches

Place a small amount of American cheese in the center of 2 mini rice cakes. If you choose, you can cook it, as you would make grilled cheese. Kids love some of the flavored rice cakes as well. This is an excellent source of calcium, complex carbohydrates, and protein.

Dippy Snacks

Kids enjoy getting a little messy while they eat, so why not make messy snacking fun for them? Cut up some fruits they like, and let the kids dip them into low-fat yogurt. Another option is to cut up some of their favorite veggies and dip them into low-fat salad dressings. This will give you a good mix of vitamins, minerals, and proteins.

S and B Smoothie

Ice cold sweet drinks are always enjoyable, especially if they're healthy. They are also better for you than cupcakes or cookies! You may substitute other fruits that your children prefer for this snack. For our example, let's use strawberries and bananas.

Freeze a sliced banana and about 10 strawberries. Once frozen, place them in a blender with an 8-ounce cup of low-fat vanilla yogurt and a cup of 100% apple juice. Blend on low speed until mixed well. Pour into a glass and enjoy. A good mixture of vitamins and minerals.

Trail Mixes

Mix together some of your children's favorite healthy foods for another nutritious snack. A great combination would be your child's preferred healthy cereal, mini-pretzels, bite size crackers, nuts, and a small amount of chocolate chips or M&Ms. Your children will love the combination, since they helped pick it. This will provide a wonderful blend of complex carbohydrates and protein.

Celery Popcorn Ship: Super Simple!

You need a piece of celery, low fat cream cheese, and some light microwave popcorn low in salt. Spread a small amount of cream cheese on the celery and then stick the pieces of popcorn on top of the cream cheese. Instant fun with a lot of crunch. Another snack high in protein, vitamins, and calcium.

Pudding Dip

Chocolate pudding can be low in fat. Use it to dip foods such as crackers and fruits for a delicious treat. This mixture will provide complex carbohydrates, protein, and calcium.

Orange Juice Ice Pops

Fill plastic cups with 100% orange juice. Place tin foil around the top and an ice cream stick through the middle of the aluminum foil, which will hold the stick in place. Place in the freezer for a few hours, then take out the ice pops and peel off the plastic cup. Pour some sprinkles on a plate and roll the orange juice ice pops around the plate so the sprinkles stick to the ice pop. The kids will enjoy a good source of potassium, vitamin C, niacin, folate, riboflavin, and magnesium; many brands of orange juice are also a good source of calcium.

Tato Snacks (also makes a great side dish)

Rinse and clean a potato, leaving on the skin. Slice it into even pieces about 1/8 inch in thickness. Place them in a toaster oven at about 350 degrees for about 15 minutes, and then flip them. Toast for another 10 minutes or until they start to blister. After they cool off, put a little ketchup on a plate, and let your children eat some healthy French fries. Season them as you think your child may enjoy them. A great idea is to prepare them the night before and place them in the refrigerator overnight. It only takes a few minutes to heat them the next day. A good source of fibers, minerals, vitamins, potassium, and complex carbohydrates.

Pudding Pops

Buy some fat-free chocolate pudding and small wafer ice cream cones. Pour the pudding into the wafer cones, dip in sprinkles, and place in freezer for 30 minutes. Provides complex carbohydrates, protein, and calcium.

Veg Pockets

Cut a piece of pita bread in half. Open the pocket and stuff with your child's favorite chopped vegetables. Sprinkle some shredded cheese on top and place it in the oven for about 2 minutes. This snack is an excellent source of vitamins and minerals. To make it more fun, have your children make the veg pockets themselves.

Pudding Pretzels

Use a brush to spread some fat-free chocolate pudding over whole wheat pretzels, and then shower them with sprinkles. Place in the freezer for an hour. Your children will love this snack supplying calcium, complex carbohydrates, and protein.

Fruit Toast

Peel a banana and place in a bowl. Use a fork to mash it all together to make a spread. Repeat the same process with strawberries. Toast a piece of bread, then spread the banana all over the toast. Top it off by spreading the strawberries over the banana for a fantastic treat. High in vitamins, minerals, potassium, and complex carbohydrates.

Frozen Grapes

Freeze grapes in a plastic bag or container for a couple of hours. They are a fun and easy snack. Grapes are full of potassium, fiber, and vitamin B.

Granola Crunch

Pour some granola into a bowl and add a few chocolate chips. Next, add 8 ounces of fat-free vanilla yogurt. Mix well and enjoy the treat. This simple snack is high in calcium, complex carbohydrates, and protein.

Whole Wheat Tortillas

Lay low-fat whole wheat tortillas on aluminum foil. Sprinkle on grated cheese and top with minced tomatoes and peppers. Place in the oven at 350 degrees for about 5 minutes and enjoy this snack high in complex carbohydrates, protein, calcium and vitamins.

Smiley Face Bread: Great for Younger Children

Take a slice of whole wheat bread and spread some low-fat cream cheese or yogurt on it. Make a smiley face on it using 2 slices of bananas for the eyes, half a strawberry for the nose, and some string cheese for the mouth. This fun snack is full of nutrition.

Hummus Snacks

Spread hummus on whole grain toast or rice crackers for a great snack. You can also dip baby carrots in the hummus for a perfect blend of crunchiness and smoothness to satisfy your child's taste buds.

Apples and Almond Butter

If your child enjoys apples, try dipping them in almond butter for a great taste. Try peanut, cashew or sunflower seed butter.

Dried Fruit

Most fruits are available in dried form. Mix with pretzels, pumpkin seeds or nuts for a healthy snack.

Rice Cakes with Nut Butter

Try rice cakes with a thin spread of almond or peanut butter or roasted tahini (a thick paste made of ground sesame seed, popular in the Middle East).

Edamame in the Pod

Edamame (soybeans) are located in the frozen food section of your supermarket. You can also purchase them already out of the shell. It is a great snack to eat sprinkled with sea salt while watching a movie. Tastes great and a high source of protein.

Wheat-Free Sunflower Crunches

This snack takes a little bit of prep, but is fun to make with the kids!

Prep Time: 10 minutes

Yield: 10–15 servings

Ingredients:

1 cup sunflower seeds, (pepitas or pumpkin seeds can be substituted, but beware, they are large!)

1/2 cup sesame seeds

1 tablespoon poppy seeds (optional)

1 tablespoon maple syrup or agave nectar

1 1/2 tablespoons olive oil

Directions:

Preheat oven to 375 degrees

Combine sunflower, sesame and poppy seeds, and then blend.

Add oil and maple syrup, and blend again.

Roll dough into several long pieces and place them on a lightly oiled baking sheet.

Bake for 15–20 minutes.

Healthy Meals You Can Prepare at Home

Breakfast Samples

Breakfast 1

Hot Oatmeal
Orange Slices
Glass of Low-Fat Milk

This breakfast includes whole grain for vitamin B, iron and fiber. Whole grains are full of natural antioxidants, and oatmeal is a good source of carbohydrates, which give the body energy, and fiber, which aids in digestion. Orange slices and other citrus fruits provide an excellent source of Vitamin C and calcium. Choose milk for calcium and Vitamin D, which helps build strong bones and teeth. Choose low-fat or non-fat dairy products for children over two years old.

Breakfast 2

Ready-To-Eat Whole Grain Cereal
Sliced Banana
Orange Juice
Glass of Low-Fat Milk

Like the oatmeal in Breakfast 1, ready-to-eat whole grain cereal is an excellent source of antioxidants, which help protect cells in the body. Choose whole grains for B vitamins, carbohydrates and fiber. The banana provides fiber and Vitamin C. Orange juice is also a great source of Vitamin C. Choose 100% fruit juice, and avoid juice drink, juice aides, or fruit punch (they all have added sugars in them). Limit the amount of 100% juice to 6 ounces per day.

Breakfast 3

Scrambled Eggs
Whole Wheat Toast
Applesauce
Glass of Low-Fat Milk

Eggs are a good source of high quality protein and B vitamins. They are also a good source of the fat-soluble vitamins A and D. Although eggs contain fat and cholesterol, they can make a tremendous contribution to a healthy diet because of the wide range of nutrients they contain. Whole grains, fruits and milk are an essential part of a healthy breakfast.

Lunch Samples

Lunch 1

Turkey Sandwich on Whole Grain Pita Bread
with Lettuce and Tomato
Glass of Low-Fat Milk

A four-ounce serving of turkey provides more than half of the daily value for protein. To avoid fat, instead of mayonnaise or butter, try mustard. Again, include whole grains. Lettuce is a good source of fiber and Vitamin C, and tomatoes are good sources of vitamins C and A, potassium and fiber. Eating a variety of vegetables and fruits, whole grains, lean protein and low-fat dairy products helps ensure a well-rounded diet that includes most of the known nutrients.

Lunch 2

Grilled Chicken Salad with Sliced Tomatoes
Top with 2 Tablespoons of Olive Oil and Vinegar
Spring Greens with Spinach
Peaches
Glass of Low-Fat Milk or Water

Like turkey, chicken is another good source of protein and an excellent source of niacin, a cancer-protective B vitamin. Choose oils like canola or olive oil to cook with instead of solid fats like butter or margarine. Spinach and other green leafy vegetables provide most of the available nutrients and are very high in Vitamin A, folate iron and Vitamin C. Fresh peaches are a fat-free treat and high in Vitamins A, C and fiber.

Lunch 3

Grilled Cheese on Whole Wheat Bread
Fresh Baby Carrots
Grape Tomatoes and Cucumbers with Ranch Dressing Dip
Fresh Plum
Glass of Low-Fat Milk

Cheese is rich in protein and vitamins and calcium, which helps build strong bones and helps fight against osteoporosis. However, limit the amount of cheese you eat since it is high in fat, and try the reduced fat or fat-free varieties. The veggies provide a colorful array of vitamins and minerals. Plums help ensure a healthy digestive system. They are loaded with vitamins and rich with the minerals potassium, phosphorus and magnesium.

Dinner Samples

Dinner 1

Tacos with Ground Turkey Breast Wrapped
in Whole-Wheat Tortillas
Top with Lettuce, Chopped Tomato and Salsa
Glass of Low-Fat Milk
Low-Fat Yogurt Topped With Blueberries

Turkey breast is a good source of lean protein and is low in saturated fat, which makes it a good food choice. Choose whole grain tortillas, but look for those that are fat-free or low in saturated fat. Low-fat yogurt with blueberries makes a nutritious and low-fat dessert and has as much calcium as one cup of milk. Blueberries are high in anti-oxidants and always make a nutritious snack.

Dinner 2

Stir-Fry Chicken and Veggies
Brown Rice
Garden Salad with Vinaigrette
2 Cookies
Glass of Low-Fat Milk

Chicken is a healthy alternative to red meat. It's low in fat and high in lean protein. However, eating chicken with the skin doubles the amount of fat and saturated fat. For this reason, chicken is best skinned before cooking. Use two tablespoons of olive oil or canola oil rather than butter or shortening. Choose brown over white rice for its nutrient value. Brown rice is a whole grain and a good source of fiber, minerals, and B vitamins.

Dinner 3

Tuna Macaroni and Cheese with Non-Fat Milk
and Reduced-Fat Cheese
Green Beans and Carrots
Glass of Low-Fat Milk
Unsweetened Applesauce Sprinkled with Cinnamon

It's best to make your own macaroni and cheese using whole grain macaroni, fat-free cheddar cheese, non-fat cottage cheese, and non-fat milk. However, if you choose boxed macaroni and cheese, use non-fat milk and fat-free butter spread. Add a can of white tuna packed in water, drained, rather than packed in oil. Tuna is a good source of protein, selenium, iron, Vitamin B_{12}, and niacin. Green beans are an excellent source of vitamin C, vitamin K (for strong bones) and manganese. Green beans are also a very good source of vitamin A and fiber. Carrots are an excellent source of antioxidant compounds, and the richest vegetable source of vitamin A. They help protect against cardiovascular disease and cancer and promote good vision. Applesauce is a favorite with children of all ages. Choose unsweetened applesauce and add cinnamon for taste. Top with raisins for iron and added texture.

CHAPTER TWELVE

To Diet or Not to Diet

Many years ago, I had the opportunity to work with a child outside of the school setting who was severely obese. I adored this child's personality and positive attitude. Her parents were worried about her health: she had recently been diagnosed with type 2 diabetes due to her extreme weight and she could not do the simple daily tasks that most of us take for granted, such as running, tying her shoes or picking up an object from the floor. Sadly, both her parents were also morbidly obese, had trouble with simple tasks, and both had diabetes as well.

This young girl was also having trouble at school. We all know how cruel and insensitive many children can be. She was being teased and having a hard time socializing; her size prohibited her from wearing trendy clothing, and her self-esteem had been shattered many times.

Over time, her parents and I teamed up on a diet and exercise plan for her. I would go to their home and work with them on their meal menus, snacks and physical activities. At times, I even helped with the grocery shopping. My initial objective was to start getting her weight down a little, and then start a very light and easy walking program. We began by adding more protein and fiber to her diet, limited portions and snacking, and had her drink more water as opposed to the sugary drinks. Most desserts were also eliminated, except for fruits. Within days, she had lost a few pounds. Presto! Now she had something positive to build on.

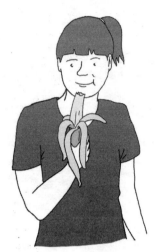

We continued to eat healthy foods, in moderation, with less snacking. We began walking together, and soon we were able to put some running and bike riding into our sessions. Be-

Sweets can come in the form of fruit instead of cookies or cake!

fore long, she knocked off 20 pounds. Her self-esteem was on the rise, and she was feeling healthier.

She didn't have to cut out any meals, nor did she lose out on important nutrients needed for proper growth and development. Simple, light exercise combined with a healthy diet made a world of difference in her life. We kept in touch after my time with her ended, and she was determined to keep moving forward. She experienced many peaks and some valleys along the way, but I always hoped for the best for her. She was an inspiration to me, and to everyone who knew her.

I tell you this story to illustrate my view that, in most cases, children should have a healthy diet, but not necessarily go on a "diet." Children's bodies are still maturing, and depriving them of calories, nutrients, vitamins, or minerals can be more dangerous than helpful to their development. Even children who are overweight can damage their bodies by depriving them of nutritious foods through skipping meals. It's important to have a game plan set up with your pediatrician if you or your doctors think your child needs to shed some weight. Here are two important principles to keep in mind:

1. **Don't Let it Become a Problem.** Try your best to avoid having your child become overweight or obese in the first place. The idea that it's easy to turn around a child's obesity in a short period of time is incorrect, and to try to do so is often dangerous. The expression "never put off to tomorrow what you can do today" definitely applies here, since, as we've already discussed, the hardest habits to break are those that begin when children are very young. Many of the unhealthy foods available to kids simply taste better to them than healthy foods, and your children will start to prefer them. Once kids are started on sugary, high calorie or high fat foods, the healthier foods will get the "yuck" response. Before you know it, the bad habit is formed. Most parents don't intend to put off taking the steps to break this bad habit, but it's all too easy to put something like this on hold until it's too late.

2. **All Things in Moderation.** Cutting out some foods completely won't necessarily give you the results you are looking for in your child. Moderation of food intake may be the smarter answer. In many cases, your pediatrician may recommend more frequent but smaller meals throughout the day. Talk to your doctor or dietitian about a game plan that may work for your child. Food higher in protein and fiber will help suppress the desire to eat, as will drinking water. If your child still feels hungry after a meal, have her take a break, relax for a while, and see if her appetite diminishes. Remember, just as your child didn't gain the weight overnight, she won't lose weight overnight. Weight loss is a slow process, where patience, motivation and determination are the keys to a positive outcome.

Sometimes, there are unique situations where a pediatrician or dietitian may start a child on a diet to lose weight. These unique cases may help save a child's life, or help them carry out daily tasks they may have trouble with, such as climbing the stairs or walking. Again, your family doctor would better be able to tell you if your child is a candidate to start dieting to lose weight.

Caloric Requirements for Kids

There is no one caloric requirement for all age groups or both genders. It all depends on body composition, activity level, types of foods eaten, overall health, and heredity. Obviously, too many calories bring the risk of a child becoming overweight, while too few calories bring the risk of poor nutrition. The best method of deciding what is right for your child is asking your pediatrician or dietitian. Figure 12.1 gives you general caloric requirements recommended by the U.S. Department of Health and Human Services and the United States Department of Agriculture. First, you must determine which activity level best describes your children's lifestyle:

Activity Level Definitions:
Sedentary: Little physical activity on a day-to-day basis.

Moderately Active: Physical activity equivalent to walking 1.5 to 3 miles per day at 3 to 4 miles per hour, plus normal day-to-day activities.

Active: Physical activity equivalent to walking more than 3 miles per day at 3 to 4 miles per hour, plus normal day-to-day activities.

Keeping it simple with children is very important in maintaining a controlled weight. As soon as things start getting complicated, a child's interest diminishes, and weight gains may occur. Here's

Figure 12. 1 *Estimated Daily Caloric Requirements*

Ages	Sedentary		Moderately Active		Active	
Gender	Boys	Girls	Boys	Girls	Boys	Girls
2–3	1000	1000	1000–1400	1000–1400	1000–1400	1000–1400
4–8	1000	1200	1400–1600	1400–1600	1600–2000	1400–1800
9–13	1800	1600	1800–2000	1600–2000	2000–2600	1800–2000
14–18	2200	1800	2400–2800	2000	2800–3200	2400

a simple formula: *If you consume more calories than you need, your body will store the extra energy as fat. If you eat fewer calories than you need, your body will burn fat to provide the extra energy.* So, the simple solution for children is to maintain a healthy balance between calories eaten and calories burned every day. The trick is to watch what they eat and make sure they remain active. Another trick to keeping the calorie count low is to monitor the liquid intake of your child. Over 20% of calories consumed by children are from liquid, so this is a key issue to look at when watching caloric intake.

I'd love to give you a Len's Top Ten list of tips for building a healthier diet for your kids, but the subject is so important—and there are so many ways to address it—that I'm going for the whole Top 40!

Len's Top 40 Tips for Healthier Eating

1. Start teaching your children at a very young age how to eat properly.
2. Cook more with olive or canola oils. Both oils are low in saturated fat and high in healthful monounsaturated fat, which can reduce the risks of cardiovascular disease.

3. Stay away from processed foods, which may be higher in calories, fat and sugar. Look for more natural, higher fiber and protein foods.

4. Reduce the amount of snacks and desserts throughout the day.

5. Reduce portion sizes at meals, especially those meals higher in fat content.

6. If your child is hungry after a meal, have him take a break from eating for a while to see if his appetite diminishes on its own.

7. Try offering your child a new (healthier) food when you think he is hungry. This is a great starting point when introducing healthier eating. But try not to introduce too many new foods at one time!

8. Do not make children eat everything on their plate if they are full. That is actually teaching them to overeat. It's important for them to know when to stop.

9. Make healthy snacking fun for kids. Make a fruit salad face. Place a strawberry for each eye, an apple for the nose, and a banana for the mouth. Your younger children will get a kick out of this.

10. Drink more water and reduce the use of sweetened drinks.

11. Stay away from simple carbohydrates, such as sugared snacks or potato chips. They are higher in fat content and will be digested quickly, causing hunger to return sooner.

12. Avoid too much red meat. Your child should not eat steak or burgers each night, and neither should you. Instead, serve lean meats such as turkey or chicken.

13. Try to substitute healthy snacks for unhealthy ones. Instead of French fries, slice up a potato and bake it in the oven or on the grill. Same great taste, less fat.

14. Don't skip meals, as it may promote more eating later on in the day.

15. Maintain a balance between your child's caloric intake and expenditure. Balance your child's intake responsibly and keep them active so those calories will not turn to fat.

16. Just because someone eats well for one week does not mean he will see immediate results when it comes to losing weight and feeling good. Keep at it, one step at a time.

17. Avoid any deep fry cooking. Instead, use the grill, roast, steam, or broil the foods. This will reduce the amount of fat in the food.

18. Serve a variety of foods. Mixing foods from various food groups is beneficial to good all-around health.

19. Don't completely deny your children junk food. Sometimes this can cause them to binge when you are not looking.

20. Try not to use food as a reward. Don't buy your children ice cream for getting straight A's on their report card. Rather, contribute to their college fund, or take them bowling.

21. If you take your children to the supermarket, be firm about what they throw into your grocery cart. Limit the unhealthy snacks.

22. Keep your children physically active, so they burn off more calories and don't have to watch their diets so closely.

23. Make healthier foods more available. If children can find the sugary snacks first, that's what they will eat first.

24. Never make eating healthy foods a punishment. Eating nutritious foods should be enjoyable, with the knowledge it can make you healthier and strong.

25. Don't mistake your child's hunger for thirst. Try giving your child water to see if the hunger goes away, especially right before a meal or bedtime.

26. Serve more high fiber foods such as fruits, vegetables, and whole grains. They will make your child feel full for a longer time, which reduces snacking.

27. Avoid foods higher in sodium (salt). Salt can cause water weight gain.

28. Learn to read product labels. Don't be afraid to put something back on the shelf at the supermarket if you don't like what's inside.
29. Feed your children more nutrient-rich foods, which include whole-grain products, vegetables, fruits, dairy products, and protein foods.
30. Try not to eliminate foods, rather, serve them in moderation.
31. Try to make sure your children snack smart throughout the day. Do not have them overindulge in a snack an hour before they have dinner.
32. Make mealtime relaxing and calm. If too much stress is brought to the table, children are more likely not to eat properly, and therefore not get the nutrients needed for proper growth and development.
33. Serve meals on a regular schedule. If you deviate times on a daily basis, you are throwing off your child's internal hunger clock.
34. Set a good example and eat healthy as a family. If your children see you eat fruits and veggies, they are more likely to join in.
35. Let your children help create the food menu. This builds an interest in what they eat, as they feel they have contributed to the decision. Work together on selecting foods that are fun, yet healthy.
36. Invite your child's friends to a meal. If you are having trouble getting your child to eat the proper foods, compromise, and allow them to bring a friend over to dinner if they eat more of the healthier foods.
37. Make meals attractive. Children respond much better to a meal that looks more appetizing than they do to a "mystery meal."
38. Teach your children to thoroughly chew their foods and to eat slowly. Eating too fast does not allow the body to properly digest food, and encourages children to overeat.

39. Avoid bringing home fast foods meals. That may be a treat once in a while when you are away from home, but must not be a daily occurrence at home.

40. Choose smart desserts for the children such as gelatin or low-fat chocolate pudding.

CHAPTER THIRTEEN

Water: The Key to Good Health

Why a whole chapter devoted just to water? Simple: drinking a glass of water is like drinking a glass of health! It is absolutely essential for life and for maintaining wellness, and a key ingredient in the recipe for keeping your kids fit and healthy. In this chapter we'll look at the importance of hydrating the body during physical activity, as well as all the general benefits of drinking water.

Water cleanses the body inside as well as outside. If a child does not drink enough liquids, his body can't eliminate waste, including bacteria and toxins, which increases the risk of infection from these agents. Cleansing the body of waste also helps increase energy, by increasing blood volume and the amount of oxygen that is carried by the blood throughout the body. Keeping the blood pumped with oxygen as it is delivered to the muscle tissue also reduces the risk of cramps during exercise.

Drinking water has a profound effect on kids' appetites. In many cases, when children are hungry, they don't reach for healthy snacks but for the chips or cookies. While water is not a food

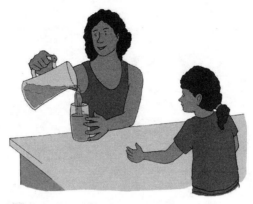

Choose water over the "liquid candy" drinks whenever possible.

replacement, it is a means to fill the stomach for a short time, which can suppress the appetite and the urge for between-meal snacks. Also, many children have a hard time differentiating between hunger and thirst, so drinking water first can take away the urge to eat entirely. It has the added benefit of raising the metabolic rate slightly and helping the body burn fat as energy more efficiently, thereby contributing to weight loss.

Water lubricates muscles, bones, joints, and other body parts, including the eyes, nose and mouth. Water speeds the conveyance of blood throughout the body, and also helps the discs of the spine maintain proper cushioning between them, reducing the lower back pain that can come with dehydration.

In addition to lubricating the food in our body to keep the digestive system running smoothly, water dilutes the stomach acids that can irritate the lower esophagus. It also assists the digestive system in breaking down foods to help supply the body with proper nutrients. These nutrients are then transported to the cells throughout the body in the blood, assisted with the intake of water in the body.

When we exercise, our body temperature goes up and water, in the form of sweat, appears on the skin as a natural cooling system. The system works best when we are properly hydrated. Keeping proper moisture in the body has the added benefit of promoting good skin health, and helps one to maintain that "healthy glow."

Water benefits the body in ways one might not even imagine. For example, many children (and adults) suffer from headaches purely from being dehydrated. In many cases, as soon as lost water is replenished and the brain re-hydrates, the headaches can disappear. The benefits of water are endless! As you can see, educating your children about its importance is imperative to maintaining all around good health.

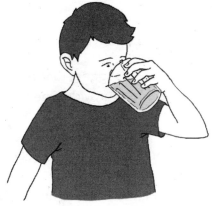

Drink sensibly. Make sure your child does not over–hydrate!

How Much Water Should a Child Drink?

There are several different theories on the proper amount of water a child should drink every day. I share them with you below, and then offer what I believe is a common sense approach to this issue. Remember, because every child is different, before you make any radical changes to your child's diet, consult your pediatrician, who will help guide you on this and all other diet decisions.

The Body Weight Approach

One way to determine the proper amount of water intake is to divide your body weight, in pounds, in half, and drink that number of ounces of water per day. For example, if you weigh 100 pounds, you should drink at least 50 ounces of water per day. Other experts suggest that drinking an amount of water in ounces equal to 1/3 of one's body weight is sufficient. Do what you feel works best for you.

The 8/8 Approach

Many experts suggest that drinking 8 eight-ounces glasses of water each day provides the right hydration. However, parents should consider other factors in determining if this is the proper amount for their children, including their level of physical activity, the local altitude, type of climate, and overall health of their children. For example, if your child is extremely active and you live in a warmer climate, it may be wiser to have more than 8 glasses a day, since there are more opportunities to lose body water.

The Input/Output Approach

The average urine output for humans is approximately 6 to 8 cups a day. This output varies among children and adults, males and female, active and non-active people, so it is hard to give a specific number that may apply to your children. Humans may lose another 2–3 cups of water a day through breathing, sweating and bowel movements. Many foods (especially fruits and vegetables) may account for 25% of your total daily fluid intake, so if you consume the remaining 75% by drinking water or other beverages each day along with your normal diet, you will typically replace the lost fluids. Of course, these numbers will vary according to age, gender, activity level, total health, diet and environment. With this method, meals and snacks that include fruits and vegetables, along with proper water intake, will keep your child sufficiently hydrated.

The Drink Throughout the Day Approach

Many health professionals believe that children should drink plenty of water throughout the day and check the color of their urine. After the initial urination of the morning, it should remain colorless throughout the remainder of the day. If the urine is yellow, (and your kids have normally functioning kidneys), it could be a sign of dehydration and that they need to drink more water.

You will probably not find one definitive answer to the question of the amount of water children need to consume daily. Here are some general guidelines that, if followed, I believe will ensure that your kids are properly hydrated:

1. Make sure they replenish lost water throughout the day. Have them take a water bottle to school, so water is always available. If your children are very active and you live in a warm climate, it's even more important to bring water along to prevent dehydration.
2. Make sure they check the color of their urine during the day. Drinking water throughout the day will assist in keeping the urine colorless.
3. Ensure that they have fruits and vegetables as snacks throughout the day, which are higher in water content than other snacks.
4. Avoid foods high in sodium to avoid water retention.
5. Teach them to drink water when away from home if they get a headache, if their body aches, or if they don't feel well.

In my view, and in the view of many health professionals, water should be the number one beverage of choice for kids, but other beverages, such as low fat milk, non-fat milk, or 100% all natural, unsweetened juice are also wise choices, in moderation. All of these drinks help to keep the body hydrated while providing nutrients for good health and growth. It's very important to choose the correct beverage for your child: studies show that some 20% of the calories obtained by children throughout the day come from liquids, so reducing the daily caloric intake from liquids alone can have an enormous positive effect on your child's weight and health. Simply swapping water for your children's favorite sugary beverages, which in many instances are nothing more than liquid candy (however "all natural" and "made with real juice" they might purport to be), can make a critical difference in their wellness.

Not only are sugary drinks bad in and of themselves, new research indicates that they may in fact stimulate the appetite. These drinks often get consumed in oversized quantities and are digested rapidly, possibly causing a child to become hungry at a faster pace. The rapid rise of the blood sugar level in the body caused by these drinks, which might initially rejuvenate the body, also leads to a rapid blood sugar level decline, causing a child to become tired, sedentary and perhaps hungry.

Parents should make wise choices when determining the amount of water their children should drink each day. Your child's pediatrician or nutritionist will provide a better perspective on the amount of liquids that will better suit your child.

One word of caution. Under normal conditions, individuals generally know how to regulate their fluid balance. It's possible, however, to over-hydrate, producing hyponatremia, a physical disorder in which there is an imbalance of water to salt in the body, which can lead to headaches, fatigue, nausea and more serious symptoms. As always, if you are uncertain, check with your doctor.

CHAPTER FOURTEEN

A Good Night's Sleep Is a Very Good Thing

A few years ago, I was giving a presentation to parents and educators about childhood obesity, and about how to motivate kids to get the most effort out of them. A physical education teacher in the audience raised his hand and described a student of his who always arrived at his early morning PE class looking disorganized and exhausted. The child frequently got hurt in his class, not because he was particularly uncoordinated, but because he was not paying attention. The teacher's attempts to get the child to reach his potential consistently failed.

This student's grades were also slipping, and it was becoming increasingly apparent that something was amiss. After some investigation, it turned out that the child was suffering from sleep deprivation, a condition that is becoming common among children all over the world.

I suggested to the teacher that he find out more about the parents' supervision of this child's sleep habits. He found out that,

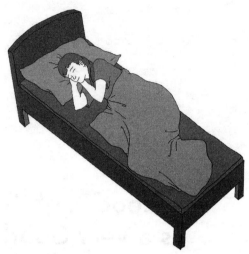

Children need the proper amount of sleep each night to be at the top of their game.

once this student's parents tucked him in at night, they never checked on him. While his parents assumed he was fast asleep, he was actually watching television with headphones, playing video games with the sound off, or playing on the computer. He even put a towel by the bottom of the door to block out any light that might pass through! Basically, he became sleep deprived, which had a significant negative impact on his academic performance, his physical health, and (perhaps not surprisingly) his temperament.

In this chapter we'll examine sleep as a significant component of good health. We'll look at the latest research on sleep requirements for growing children and adolescents, as well as how these requirements may differ among individual children. You'll find strategies for helping your child get adequate rest, including fun and easy ways to establish age-appropriate nighttime routines. We'll also discuss the benefits of sleep, as well as the effects of sleep deprivations on the human body.

How Much Sleep Is Needed?

There is no definitive amount of sleep children should have each night, as individual differences play a key role in what's needed. But most experts agree that many children, as well as adults, are not getting the recommended amount of sleep for good health and optimal performance. Figure 14.1 shows the recommended amounts of sleep for children of various ages. If your child falls within these guidelines for sleep each night, and is able to function properly on a daily basis, then he is getting adequate sleep.

Figure 14.1 *Recommended Amounts of Sleep for Children (Actual numbers may vary depending on individual differences)*

Infants: 14–16 hours of sleep per day

Toddlers: 12–14 hours of sleep per day

Ages 3–5: 11–13 hours of sleep per day

Ages 5–12: 10–11 hours of sleep per day

Ages 12–14: 9–10 hours of sleep per day

Ages 14–18: 8–9 hours of sleep per day

The Stages of Sleep

Children experience four basic stages of sleep each night. They are:

Stage 1. Stage 1 is considered a transition period between wakefulness and sleep. This is light sleep, when children drift in and out of sleep and can be awakened easily. In this stage, the eyes roll slowly and muscle activity slows down. This stage lasts only a few minutes.

Stage 2. In this stage, eye movement stops while heart rate, temperature, and breathing begin to slow down. It can last between 5 and 15 minutes, and during this period the brain begins to produce bursts of rapid, rhythmic brain wave activity.

Stage 3. Stage 3 is sometimes called "deep sleep" or "delta sleep" during which children make the conversion from a light sleep to a deep sleep. Delta brain waves (slow brain waves) begin to surface in this stage, heart and respiration rates become more regular, and it can be very difficult to wake someone up during this stage. Sleep talking, sleep walking, and night terrors tend to happen in this stage of sleep.

REM. REM sleep gets its name from the rapid eye movement that takes place during this stage, along with increased brain activity and an increased respiration rate. Brain waves during this stage increase to levels similar to when a person is awake, the heart rate increases and blood pressure rises. This is the time when most dreams occur. Most people experience three to five intervals of REM sleep each night.

The Benefits of Sleep

- **Sleep helps to rest the body.** Without sleep, our bodies cannot recharge for the next day. As you read further, you'll see how the body works hard for you while you sleep.
- **Sleep helps breathing to slow down at nighttime.** This is important, because during the day your heart pumps faster, causing you to breathe harder. A good night's sleep helps level off rapid breathing, putting your body in a more relaxed mode, allowing you to put stress or anxiety away for many hours.
- **Sleep slows the heart rate.** In stressful situations, the heart will beat much faster, which frequently occurs during the day. A consistently rapid heart rate can cause other problems if not controlled or reduced. A good night's sleep will help slow down the heart, allowing it to recuperate.

- **Sleep helps repair damaged cells, which help kids grow.** When asleep, the body is performing repair work that it can't complete during the time it is awake. It will regenerate damaged cells, repair tissue, and undergo an overall renewal process for all bodily functions, which prepares you for all the challenges of the coming day.
- **Sleep helps the body control appetite.** Research suggests that getting enough sleep keeps hormone levels that are related to appetite stable, helping you to feel satisfied and full after you eat. Conversely, sleep deprivation keeps these hormone levels lower, which may cause you to feel hungry after you complete a meal. Sleep also helps you retain more energy from the foods you have eaten which in turn will give you more energy to burn during the following day.
- **Sleep helps improve cognitive skills and concentration.** While sleeping, the brain is busy rejuvenating neurons so that it may continue to function well. A sleep-deprived child can have problems with broken concentration and clumsiness.
- **Sleep can help improve memory.** Sleep is like food for your brain. Sleep helps to repair and rejuvenate your memory processes, and stimulate overall growth and development.
- **Sleep fights depression.** Sleep influences many of the chemicals in your body, such as serotonin, a brain chemical that gives us self-confidence and an all-around good feeling. People with low serotonin levels are prone to suffer from depressive moods.
- When your body is sleep deprived, it goes into a state of stress. This causes a rise in blood pressure, which increases the risk for heart attacks and strokes. High levels of stress can also impact your ability to fall asleep at night.
- **Sleep helps us look and feel better.** In many cases, children who don't get enough sleep don't look healthy, with dark circles under the eyes, a pale complexion, and a lack of that "healthy glow."

- **Proper sleep can help prevent illnesses.** Sleep affects the human body's ability to regulate insulin levels and to metabolize glucose effectively. Not only does insulin control blood sugar, but it also promotes fat storage, which can make weight loss more difficult. Getting the proper amounts of sleep can help prevent some mental illnesses. Sleep deprivation has been known to cause mood swings, making individuals irritable and combative. A lack of sleep has been associated with creating blood pressure and cholesterol problems, both of which are known risk factors for heart disease and stroke. Improper sleep habits have been associated with obesity. Children who stay up later have more time to become hungry and to eat.

Aa lack of sleep elevates materials in the blood that are responsible for increasing inflammation in the body, which has recently been determined to be a major risk factor for heart disease, cancer, stroke, and diabetes. Also, researchers have found that several days of sleep deprivation results in the development of inattention and hyperactive symptoms in children who never displayed them before. When children are sleepy, they often become overly active due to an increase in the production of adrenaline by the body. Some children can be mistaken for being hyperactive when the real problem is that they habitually lack enough sleep. The same applies to performance: kids are able to reach their potential for a short while, then dip to a lesser performance. At the very least, children who get low amounts of sleep can be prone to tantrums and a poor attitude.

Nighttime Routines

Since kids need consistent sleep, a routine is very helpful in making sure they get the sleep they need. Here are some tips to ensure healthy sleeping habits:

- **Be consistent.** It's very important for parents to be firm about getting their children into bed at a regular time each night. Once you enforce a routine, your children will fall into a comfort zone, and should fall asleep within a reasonable time.
- **Avoid heavy exercise before bedtime.** Physical activity before bedtime is sometimes the culprit for your child's inability to sleep. Activity keeps the body in a more energetic state and less inclined to slow down, as the heart rate becomes elevated along with the energy level. In some studies, light exercise such as yoga and walking have been shown to help sleep, as they release tension without over-stimulating the body. As stated previously, individual differences may apply when it comes to your child's sleep patterns. Use your judgment based on your child's needs when determining how much activity before bedtime is appropriate.
- **Read before bed.** Have your children read before bedtime, or read a book to them if they are not able to read on their own. The session should not be too long, as you do not want children to associate bedtime with anything other than sleep. Have your children read books that are not too stimulating, such as short stories or spiritual books. In many cases, parents should only allow their children to read at their desk in their room, so the bed will be associated only with sleeping. Many parents have their older children relax by writing in a personal journal before bedtime.
- **Avoid technology in bed.** Television, movies, cell phones, and video games are stimulating and make it harder for your children to fall asleep.
- **Listen to soft music.** Relaxing and soft sounds before bedtime, such as classical music, have a tranquilizing effect on many children. Other music genres may be too stimulating for children to listen to at night, causing them to have trouble falling asleep. Some people find nature sounds, such as ocean waves, rainfall or crickets in the forest to be soothing.

- **Alert your child that bedtime is coming.** If you just tell your children to stop what they are doing and get to bed, most likely you will receive some resistance. It's a good idea to give your children a warning that bedtime is coming. Follow the 30/15/5/2 rule: give them a warning at 30 minutes, 15 minutes, 5 minutes, and then 2 minutes before bedtime. This allows them to close any existing projects they may be working on at the time.
- **Bathe before bedtime.** Taking a warm bath before bed is very relaxing, and puts the body and mind in a relaxing state. Make sure the water is neither too hot nor too cold, as temperature extremes can be stressful for the body, which could interfere with sleep.
- **Wear comfortable pajamas.** Many children can't fall asleep because their bed attire is uncomfortable. Avoid tight clothing that makes a child feel restricted.
- **Reduce the light in the room.** The human brain becomes stimulated when exposed to light, so darkness helps with sleeping. A low watt nightlight will not affect a child's sleep pattern as much as a bright light from other parts of the house.
- **Avoid simple carbohydrates (sugars) and caffeine before bed.** Some foods high in sugar will prevent your child from falling asleep, and wake him up during the night. Snacks that are good at bedtime include warm milk, light fruit, yogurt, cheese and crackers, and non-sugared cereal. Children should also avoid foods with caffeine at bedtime, since caffeine is a stimulant.
- **Limit beverages before bed.** Too much liquid before bed may cause children to wake up more frequently to use the bathroom.
- **Make lists.** If your child is worried about what to do tomorrow, have her make a "to do" list that puts her mind at ease.
- **Wake up at a same time each day.** Getting up at a regular time is just as important as getting to bed at a regular time.

- **Go to the bathroom before bed.** A great rule of thumb is to always have your children visit the bathroom before bedtime, even if they say they do not have to use it. This will help eliminate the early morning wakeup to empty the bladder.
- **Massage your children.** Massage has a soothing and calming effect on most children. Simple stroking around the hairline area of the head will put them into that "sleep zone."
- **Don't be afraid to experiment.** Just as your child may believe in the tooth fairy, the power of thought may help him relax and go to sleep. For example, if your child is having trouble sleeping, ask him to put on socks to sleep. Tell him it used to work for you as a child.

Coping with Sleep Disorders

You may find that your child cannot fall asleep at night or has trouble sleeping and nothing you try helps. It's possible that your child has a common sleep disorder. Many of these problems are associated with poor sleep habits or with anxiety about falling asleep. For most young children, bedtime is a time of separation from their parents, which many kids will try to prevent from occurring. It may be a good idea to visit your child's pediatrician for a full checkup, to look for solutions to some common sleep disorders your child may experience.

Sleepwalking

Most children who sleepwalk do not suffer from emotional problems, nor do they need any treatment. But sleepwalking can be dangerous as well as disruptive. It's important to monitor your child at night as best as you can. Try to remove dangerous objects around the house that he may accidentally touch, and make sure all windows and doors are locked. Your child may get out of bed and walk around the room or the house looking very dazed, clumsy and completely disorientated. You may try to talk with him, but he probably will not acknowledge you. When you find your child sleepwalking, gently guide him back to bed. You should not yell, shake, or wake your child up. Sleepwalking episodes tend to be worse if children are sleep deprived or have irregular sleep schedules. At times, these episodes could be manifestations of other underlying sleep disorders.

Sleep Talking

Sleep talking refers to talking out loud in one's sleep. It varies in volume, ranging from simple sounds to long speeches, and can occur many times during the night. Sleep talking is harmless and very common among young children, and most will outgrow it by adolescence.

Bed Wetting

Most children do not wet the bed on purpose. Bed-wetting occurs for many reasons, such as genetic factors, stress, trouble waking up at night, or even a urinary tract infection. Millions of children wet the bed every night. It is a quite embarrassing scenario for children to deal with, and most try to keep it a secret. It's important to teach your child that he will eventually outgrow it, and realize he is not alone with this common issue. It is also important to teach your child to empty his bladder before bed, and to avoid drinking too much after dinner. Parents should never punish their children after a bed wetting episode.

Childhood Insomnia

Like their parents, children with insomnia either have trouble going to sleep, staying asleep, or do not feel rested from what should be a normal amount of sleep time. Some symptoms of childhood insomnia are feeling tired throughout the day, irritability, hyperactivity, depression, hostility, poor memory, aggressiveness and a decreased attention span. In many cases, insomnia can be addressed by having your children go to bed a little earlier, as their bedtime may be too late for their age. Your children's pediatrician may be able to help.

Night Terrors and Nightmares

Many parents consider night terrors and nightmares to be the same, but in fact they are very different. Generally, night terrors happen to children (mostly males) approximately ages 4 to 12, while nightmares happen to people of any age or gender. With night terrors, most children do not remember what happened, while with a nightmare, there is some memory of the incident. With a night terror, while still asleep the child suddenly sits upright and screams, and may be sweating and breathing fast. His pupils may appear larger, and he can remain asleep with his eyes wide open. With a nightmare, the child can wake up from fear and anxiety. In both cases, the parents can try to find out what is causing the fear or anxiety and try to change it. For night terrors, it is recommended that your home be made safe at night, with doors and windows locked and dangerous objects safely put away.

Obstructive Sleep Apnea

Obstructive sleep apnea is thought to affect one to three percent of children. It's characterized by recurring episodes of upper airway obstruction that occur during sleep, possibly due to enlarged tonsils or the tongue and excess tissue in the airway. Symptoms include snoring, difficulty breathing during sleep, excessive sleepiness during the day and impaired performance in school. It can also cause hyperactivity or attention deficit. Studies show many children misdiagnosed with ADHD started behaving normally after underlying sleep apnea is treated appropriately.

Sleep: A Powerful Friend

Children need to understand that sleep is a powerful friend that helps them be the best they can be. It helps them to feel healthy, fight colds, feel stronger, do better in school, feel more alert and look great. And not only that, it's free! You don't have to shop for it, borrow it or spend money on it. All you need to do is make time for it. Teach your children to remember the importance of sleep by this simple acronym (Figure 14.2).

Figure 14.2 *The Importance of Sleep: a Simple Reminder*

S = Stress is reduced

L = Learning improves

E = Energizes the body

E = Elevates your awareness

P = Prevents sickness

Afterword

Looking Ahead

I hope this book has shown you that it's never too late to educate your children on the countless benefits of leading a healthy lifestyle. You've learned the fundamentals of establishing and maintaining their health, of breaking bad habits and instilling good ones, and of programs that you can do at home and elsewhere that will make your children active participants in their own success.

Envision these results for your kids: they are better rested and more motivated. They have a greater sense of self-esteem. They're less prone to injury. They are even doing better in school because they are spending less time with video games and, since they are fit, they're more alert and focused.

Now envision the results for yourself: you are no longer so worried about your children's well being, because you can see them doing better and taking an interest. You share in their pride with every positive step. And you may even be healthier yourself, since you're leading by example and participating with them as much as you can in their exercise and healthy eating.

If you've waited until you finished reading this book to start putting these ideas into action, don't wait any longer. Get started now for your children's sake. With this information, and a commitment to help your kids, you can do it. You *can* lead by example. You *can* make a concrete, continuing impact on the health of your children. You and your kids *can* partner in an enjoyable, positive way to ensure their health and well being.

There is no doubt that we are facing an epidemic of poor physical fitness in children. Many health professionals state that this could be the first generation of children whose life expectancy could be lower than that of their parents. It's my firm belief that it is in our power to turn this trend around! As a parent, you are the "front line" in the fight to regain our children's health. It's important for you to keep up the rewarding work of laying the foundation for their healthy future.

And, really, what could be a greater reward for a parent than knowing his or her children are ready, willing and able to lead lives blessed with good health?

Index

About the Author

Len Saunders graduated with honors from the University of Bridgeport in Connecticut, majoring in Physical Education, and was voted "outstanding senior" by his graduating class. He went on to receive a Master's degree in Exercise Physiology from Montclair State University in New Jersey.

Len has been involved in children's health and fitness for over 25 years and has won awards for his contribution to children's health and fitness at the local, state, and national levels. He has been a guest speaker at universities and state and national conventions, and has served as a consultant to The President's Council on Physical Fitness and Sports. Most recently, he was appointed an American Heart Association spokesperson on childhood obesity and fitness.

Len's contribution to children's fitness has reached millions of children and their parents through his fitness programs Project ACES and Project PACES, his contributions to national magazines including *Muscle & Fitness* and Human Kinetics Publishing, and through his work as a consultant for *Sports Illustrated for Kids*. *Ladies Home Journal* has stated that "nobody is more committed to children's fitness than Len Saunders."

Habit-Busting Contract

I, _____ promise to end my bad habit of _____. I want to lead a healthy lifestyle.

(child's name)   (name of habit)

If the contract is broken, I know my family will work together on stopping my bad habit.

I understand that I am on the honor system. This means my parents cannot monitor my life 24 hours a day, and I will try to fulfill my end of this contract when they are not around.

I understand that my parents care about me, and want me to stop this bad habit because they love me.

_____
Date Signed

_____
Child's Signature

_____
Parent's Signature

From *Keeping Kids Fit* by Len Saunders

Downtime-from-Online Contract

I, _____ , promise to reduce my time using technology for fun and spend more time exercising and
     (child's name)

playing. This promise is made to _____ , to show them that I want to stay healthy and active.
                                      (parents' names)

If I break this contract, I know that my family and I will work together on making sure I stick with the program.

I understand that I am on the honor system. This means my parents cannot monitor my life 24 hours a day, so I
will try to keep up my end of this contract when I am not with them.

I understand that my parents care about me, and want me to reduce my technology time because they love me.

_____
Date Signed

_____
Child's Signature

_____
Parent's Signature

From *Keeping Kids Fit* by Len Saunders